Beginning GOLF

2nd Edition

By Robert Gensemer

Edinboro University of Pennsylvania

Morton Publishing Company

925 W. Kenyon Avenue, Unit 12
Englewood, Colorado 80110

Preface

The ball lies there, serenely helpless, against a backdrop of green. Your club sends the inert ball into a gravity-defying perfect flight, then to arc into a parabolic weightless fall and a rolling finish at its appointed destination. This is one of the most pleasurable moments in all sporting endeavors.

It is easy to be fascinated by this game.

But to become consistently good at golf takes time. Skill is not acquired by birthright alone. It evolves through guided practice. Even top level players had to give countless hours to developing their aptitudes. They, too, had to evolve. And during the evolution, everyone who takes up the game goes through the phases of dribbling the ball nine feet, or spinning the ball into the trees, or cuffing it 45 degrees left of target.

In the beginning it could be discouraging. The game tends to impose early disappointments on its apprentices. It's not easy to get good at golf. It's not an easy game.

Eventually, however, everything will coalesce.

This book will help. It is designed to assist all who read it to become a skilled, perceptive, self-appraising player. Prior experience is not a prerequisite. The chapters herein are for everyone.

The dialogue is not excessively detailed, as golf-talk often becomes. The considerations move from the basics of the swing to more specific matters such as hitting for power, or how to putt effectively, or how go get out of a sand trap. Most chapters end with condensed "reminders" about the techniques described and a "problem solving" section which tells of how to correct flaws.

These pages contain useful information. So do books on flying an airplane. But neither is enough, without practice and instruction, to ensure a successful performance.

Acknowledgments

A couple of dozen different players have been photographically captured for the pages of this book. Several, however, deserve particular mention for their giving of extended time for the camera: Heidi Harrington, Lance Ledbetter, Jenny Young, Tim Cook, and a dedicated thanks to Michéle and Donnica Gensemer. Half of the photos were taken by John Youngblunt. The rest are by the author. Gratitude is extended to the management of the following golf courses, who graciously allowed the taking of photographs on their site: Heather Ridge and Wellshire Golf Course in Denver, Colorado, Culbertson Hills in Edinboro, Pennsylvania, and Riverside in Cambridge Springs, Pennsylvania. Steve Carney, pro at Riverside, provided a valuable critique of the manuscript.

Contents

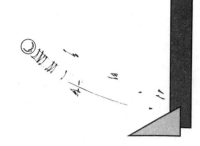

The Game

It is often suggested that golf has a benign spiritual quality, holding its participants in thrall by forces of entrancement only dimly understood. There can be an encompassing captivity of the psyche that is known only by those who play. It excites and it pleases. It challenges and it exhilarates. It wins a player's allegiance easily, often for a lifetime.

The game emerges from basic values. To hit is the very essence of golfing pleasure. Then the enlivening walk from shot to shot. And finally to sink into each pocket of the earth. On all that land where golf is played, subtle powers of energy and mystique converge. The game is paced to concentrate the mind, and complex to require all of one's mental devising and physical prowess. The feel of the club in the hands and the crystalline view of the pastoral setting — this is a place to practice fascination.

To play golf is to need good sense and an occasional gamble. It requires steadiness of purpose and physique. It asks for long shots and delicate shots; power and a deft hand; calm nerves and a certain flamboyance.

Golf has a gravity all its own. There is a transcendental veneration within the elements of the game. It's easy to be hypnotized — not hypnotized in the sense of a loss of consciousness, but rather in the regard of intrigue. It happens readily, afflicting the great majority who play.

THE SCENE

Golf is a journey — a prescribed excursion with eighteen stopovers that begins and ends at essentially the same place. So they call it a "round" of golf.

Each of the eighteen holes in a round of golf has a designated starting point — an area of turf called a **tee**, which also is the term designating the peg upon which the ball is usually placed for the first shot of the hole.

1

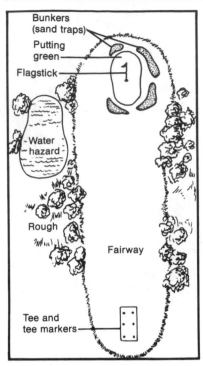

Bunkers
(sand traps)

Putting
green

Flagstick

Water
hazard

Rough

Fairway

Tee and
tee markers

There are often three sets of markers on the tee area. Furthest back (most distant from the hole) is the pro tee, so called because it must be used by professional players, and anyone else wanting to take the longest route to the hole. The middle markers designate the men's tee, and in front is the ladies' tee.

From the tee the ball is hit, hopefully, into the **fairway**, that being the long and narrow (**too** narrow, it often seems) expanse of cropped grass that is intended to be the area of play between the tee and the hole. But another destiny sometimes awaits, as the ball instead finds its way into the **rough**, where grass and weeds are left to grow freely and trees may block the passage. Or the ball plunks into a **bunker**, where instead of sod there is sand.

Final destination is the **green**, where a flagstick marks the hole. It's an emerald isle of grass often set amidst a sea of bunkers. Once on the green, the game miniaturizes to putting.

Distance from tee to green? It varies. It could be as short as 125 yards, or more than 500 yards. Total distance for the entire course? Usually about 6,500 to 6,700 yards.

Each hole has a **par**, which is the score a good player should achieve on that hole. It's either three, four, or five for the hole, and normally is a total of seventy-two for the eighteen holes. Do players accomplish that? Most do not. About ninety percent of the people who play do not consistently score better than **bogey** golf, which is an average of one stroke over par for each hole, or ninety for the round. The other players, with higher scores, have more total pleasure of the hit.

▎• THE INSTRUMENTS OF PLAY

Golf clubs are often held accountable for poor shots. But in fact they are refined, accurately balanced, optimally designed implements, well suited for their purpose.

Other games afford the player only one hitting device (as in tennis, badminton, racquetball, etc.). But the golfer is granted an array of instruments, which adds the element of selecting the appropriate club for each given situation. There could be so many choices that the rules, perhaps partly in regard for a golfer's shoulder, which is often asked to bear the weight of a bag of clubs, forbid carrying more than fourteen at a time.

The No. 1 wood, commonly called the **driver**, provides the most distance of all the clubs, and the **woods** in general, because of their larger mass, offer more distance than the **irons**. Paradoxically, the woods today are routinely constructed entirely of metal, without wood.

Each club has a **loft**, that being the degree to which its hitting face tilts back from the vertical. The relationship is: The higher the number of the club, the greater its loft; and the greater the loft, the higher the trajectory it will give to a struck ball.

The golfer who owns a complete set of clubs will likely carry a driver, a couple of other woods, irons 3 or 4 through 9, a pitching wedge, a sand wedge, and a putter. A **starter** set usually consists of Nos. 1 and 3 woods, Nos. 3, 5, 7, and 9 irons, and a putter.

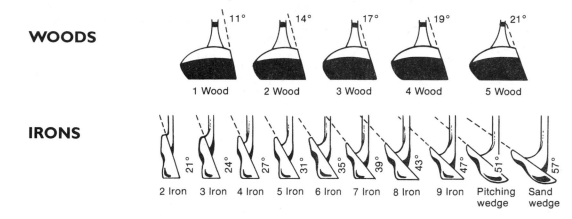

WOODS

1 Wood   2 Wood   3 Wood   4 Wood   5 Wood

IRONS

2 Iron 3 Iron 4 Iron 5 Iron 6 Iron 7 Iron 8 Iron 9 Iron Pitching Sand
wedge wedge

THE PLAYER

Then there is the golfer, who is responsible for making the clubs do what they are designed to do. It's a direct task of muscular mechanics. There is no stress of time, since the ball simply lies there serenely waiting to be hit. So the golfer need not be pressured into swatting the thing until every physical and mental resource is in proper readiness.

But the swing must be a work of precision, for golf is a finite game and the ball is unforgiving. In tennis, by comparison, if a ball is hit a half-inch away from the exact center of the racket, it doesn't really matter. But strike a golf ball a half-inch from the center of the clubhead and the results could be devastating.

So it can be concluded: golf is not an easy game to master, and for that reason it may frighten some people away. But there is also no doubt that a well-coordinated, functional swing can be achieved by anyone having enough muscle control to drive a car. Faulty swings are often the product of misunderstanding or misinterpretation

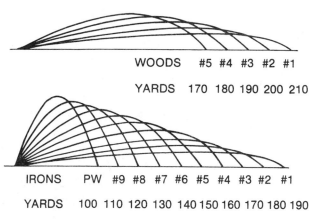

WOODS   #5 #4 #3 #2 #1

YARDS   170 180 190 200 210

IRONS   PW #9 #8 #7 #6 #5 #4 #3 #2 #1

YARDS   100 110 120 130 140 150 160 170 180 190

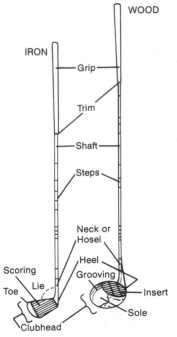

rather than a lack of ability. The brain, in effect, gives the body wrong instructions. Therefore the good news is that golf can readily be learned through a logical chain of events, properly ordered, and in fact an acceptable command of the game is not nearly so complicated as it is often made to seem.

PARALYSIS BY ANALYSIS

In all of sports, perhaps no other athletic act has been so thoroughly analyzed as the golf swing. As a result, there is a full storehouse of instructional information widely available. Consequently, an aspiring golfer can easily become overwhelmed with an endless barrage of suggestions about the turpitudes lurking in the subtle bend of an elbow, or the turn of a wrist, or the lift of a heel. It tends to clutter rather than clarify.

The brain has only a given amount of thinking room. It cannot effectively entertain an unlimited volume of thoughts about the swing while at the same time trying to organize the vast galaxy of neural affairs that will order the muscles into a productive movement. The result would be tight muscles and a hampered swing. So the best method is often the simplest — and surprisingly **all** that is needed. It makes for an agreeable harmony of mind and body, and a much higher probability of generating an efficient style of play.

THERE ARE NO SECRETS

Best of all, there are no gimmicks, no mysteries, no esoteric methods to the development of effective playing technique. Nothing is confidential or classified. There are no secrets used by professional players but never divulged to the public. Nor does any one person know something about golf that no one else knows. Instead, everything about the game is unabashedly straightforward. The choreography of a sound swing is a study of basic motion, with variations on the single theme of rhythm.

The foundation is in the absolute and definable laws of physics. The body is a collection of levers. The club is also a lever. So the definition of effective hitting can be found in the science of matter and motion. Accordingly, it becomes possible to describe the irreducible absolutes of what the brain must tell its skeletal levers to do so the ball can be sent to a predetermined place. In the final analysis it makes the game infinitely comprehendable. The framework is in the mechanics of motion, tempered to a measureless extent by that fine human quality of being able to give timing and rhythm to a prescribed movement.

Effective Technique

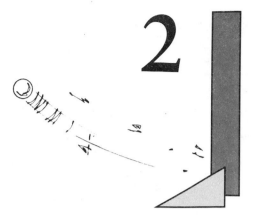

The recurring theme of golf is rhythm. It is first seen on the tee, with the overtly dynamic act of driving the ball for distance. But it is also noticed on the putting green, where a gentle tap of the ball sends it home. And it is the central ingredient of every shot in-between.

Watch the better players. Rhythm is evident in each strike of the ball. They play with a flair that shows in freedom of movement and flamboyance of style.

- Better players **look** different. They appear more relaxed, yet their swing is alive, energetic, and when needed, explosive.

- They are **poised**, in full command of their physical and mental resources.

- The club seems to be a **part** of them — a literal extension of their physical self.

- Every stroke is **fluid** — not segmented into mechanical parts, but a continuous, rhythmical, flowing motion.

- They hit the ball **decisively**, not passively nor apprehensively.

- They **enjoy** the free expression of hitting the ball. They are physically, as well as mentally, stimulated by the challenge of the game.

In total perspective, to play golf well requires a compatible blend of body and mind. It is physical aptitude, acquired through well-planned rehearsal, along with the mental willingness to experiment and the psychological readiness to hit without restraint. When all is in harmony, the ball jumps off the club with an invigorating liveliness and the game is an energizer.

5

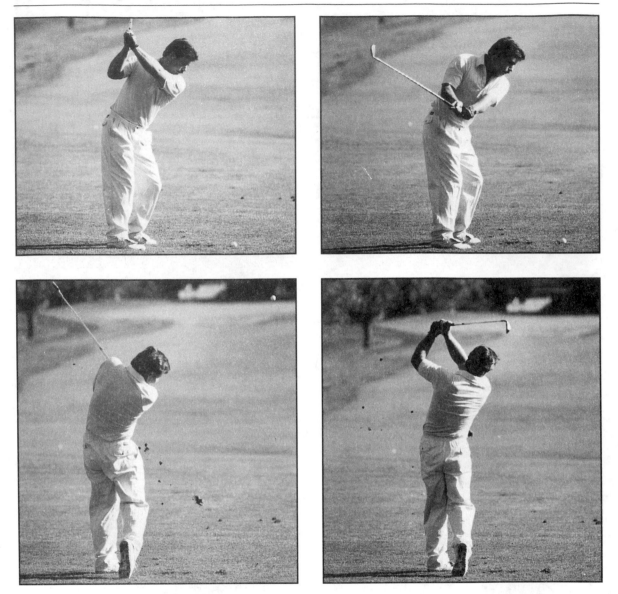

⌐. THE SWING

Although the skills of golf are based on mechanics, the game cannot be played with machine-like insensitivity. It requires physical freedom, spontaneously granted from mind to body. The strokes must have **flow**. The body needs full sanction to be unconstrained.

It begins with a deliberate, comfortable setup to the ball in preparation for the swing. When all is in readiness, there is a smooth pivot of the

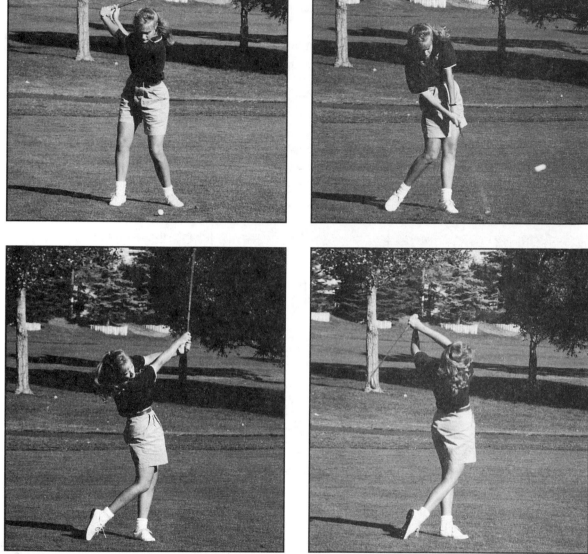

body into a coiled backswing, followed by a recoiling downswing for a responsive and affirmative strike of the ball, finishing with a free-flowing follow-through. Every stroke, whether it be intended for long distance or only short length, has a careful preparation, an unhurried start, a solid middle, and an unrestrained finish. It makes for a fluid, continuous motion of wind and unwind. The sensation is one of **gliding** through the stroke — **allowing** the body to hit rather than **forcing** it through the swing. It is effortless energy in motion.

1. COMING TO GRIPS

Everything should be in proper readiness before beginning each swing. And the first part of swing preparation is to assume a reliable grip. A sound grip is of vital importance because it must: (1) meld the hands into operating as a unit, (2) hold the face of the club firm against the concussion of impact, and (3) dependably send the clubface squarely into the ball.

The basic objective is to create a unifying of the hands. Start by setting the club into your open left hand. Run its handle across your palm at a diagonal, in particular sensing two contact points: one as upward pressure at the base of your first finger, the other as downward pressure under the heel of your hand. Be careful not to let the handle slip over the heel to rest against the base of your thumb. Now fold your hand around the handle. Feel sturdiness in your last three fingers, for they must keep the club steady at impact. Push your thumb down the club — make it a "long thumb."

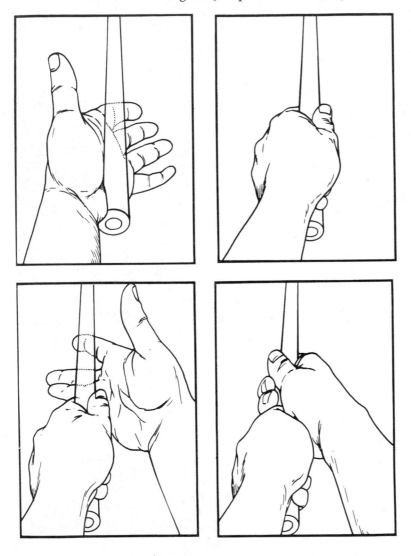

The right hand finds the club in more of a finger grip. Slide the base of your middle two fingers under the club, snugged up against your left hand. Now close your hand, laying the lifeline of your palm directly over your left thumb. Keep your right thumb askew to the left of the handle, and extend your first finger slightly in a "trigger finger" fashion under the club where it will provide a considerable lever advantage in the swing.

⌊. GRIP VARIATIONS

Overlapping Grip

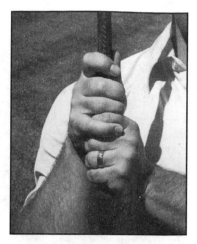

The grip just described is the overlapping grip, so called because the small finger of the right hand overlies the first finger of the left hand. It's the most widely used grip among the pros, making for a fine unity of the hands by offering feel, suppleness, and precision for the swing. Be cautious not to grasp the club too tightly, which would destroy rhythm and timing in the swing. And whichever style of grip you eventually choose, keep the **back** of the left hand and the **palm** of the right hand (along with the clubface) square to the target as you set up to the ball.

Interlocking Grip

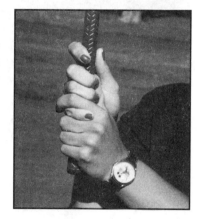

Some players prefer an interlocking grip, in which the little finger of the right hand and first finger of the left hand are actually cinched around each other. This may provide the user with a greater sense of strength and a better feel of both hands blending together as one. It may thus be easier to learn to whip the clubhead into the ball with this grip, for the two hands are automatically bonded into working together. For any grip, keep the palms **facing each other**.

Ten-Finger Grip

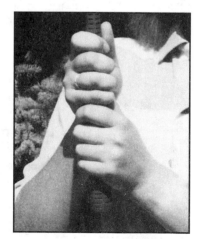

Otherwise called the baseball grip, the little finger of the right hand does not overlap or interlock, but instead wraps around the handle as do the other fingers. It's said to be for players with small hands, or anyone who likes the feel of all fingers directly on the club. The disadvantage is a tendency to let the hands operate independently. So snug your hands close together, and for any grip keep the club primarily in the **fingers** of the right hand to promote maximum "touch" or "feel."

▌• FIND A PROPER SETUP

Accurate alignment at address to the ball will enable you to swing the club along a direct path to the target. Set your aim by first standing behind the ball, then sight a definite target in the dis-

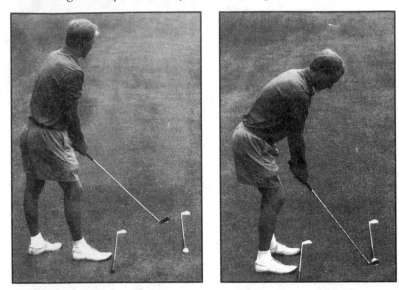

tance. Draw an imaginary line — the target line — from the ball to the chosen point of aim. Now step up to the ball. Align your feet, knees, hips, and shoulders **with the target line**. A sequence for acquiring this stance is to place the clubhead squarely behind the ball, set the back foot into position, and then station the front foot.

The finished position can be checked by placing a

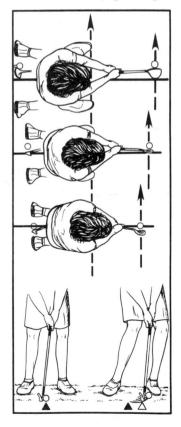

club across your toes. It should be parallel with another club, placed in front of the ball, to represent the target line. Keep your body, especially your shoulders, lateral with the target line.

Give some flex to your knees, and lower your seat several inches, as if you were about to sit on a bar stool. Let your arms hang naturally, extended without strain, toward the ball. Have the right elbow bent a bit to correctly seat the right shoulder lower than the left. Hold the clubface absolutely square to the target. Distribute your weight evenly, not only between both feet, but also between toes and heels.

▌• POSITION THE BALL PROPERLY

Tradition has it that for a driver the setup should find the ball opposite a point an inch or two inside the left heel, as schematically illustrated here in the top figure. For the middle irons the ball would be more toward the center of the stance, but still slightly forward, while the short irons have the ball positioned in the middle of the feet.

However, a major consideration is the characteristics of a full swing. The illustration on page 10 (bottom left) shows a setup with the ball midway between both feet, presumably where the club will reach the lowest point of the arc during the swing. But when a swing is taken with the intent of hitting for good distance, the bottom of the swing arc moves quite naturally forward. Therefore the ball should be placed more in relation to the strength of the ensuing swing rather than to the particular club being used. Consequently the setup should have the ball forward in the stance when wanting to hit hard, and more toward the middle when distance is less of an objective. Some pro players keep the ball forward, off the inside of the left heel, for **all** shots. In any case, place it where you'll hit the ball, not the turf.

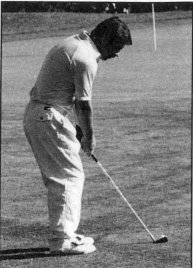

BE NATURAL; STAY RELAXED

In your setup, never feel like you're straining to reach out for the ball. From your stance of slightly flexed knees and slumped shoulders, let your arms hang freely. This will find your hands below an imaginary line running from your shoulders to the ball. The feeling in your body should be one of being "settled down" rather than leaning forward. Don't exaggerate any aspect of your posture. Everything should be natural, unforced. The whole attitude should suggest relaxation. Slacken any tension out of your body. Consciously untie your muscles. Ease your grip. Feel like you're at rest, yet alive and energetic.

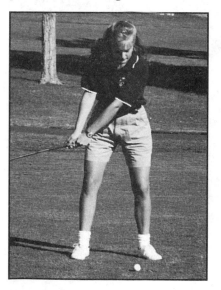

USE A UNIT TAKEAWAY

When everything is in readiness, start the club back with a whole-unit turn of the body. Begin the backswing with arms, shoulders, hips all turning together. Start back in one piece. Take the club **straight back** from the ball, without breaking the wrists, keeping the clubface flush to the ball, until your body turn naturally takes the club inside the target line. This makes your shoulders rotate from the very beginning. Start smoothly and deliberately. Keep your left arm and club in the same relationship they had at address, then allow the arm to bend slightly and the wrists to hinge naturally as the backswing reaches completion.

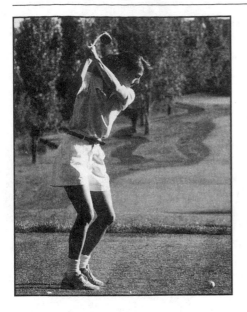

▙● KEEP A STEADY HEAD

Think of your head as the hub of a wheel, your arms as the spokes, and your spine as the axle. Swing by turning your arm-spokes around your spine-axle while holding your head-hub steady. Keeping your head in one place during the swing will eliminate body sway, or pulling away from the ball, and will cancel a whole series of other flaws. So give your head nothing to do except three things it was designed for: thinking, looking, listening. Let it think about staying in one place. Let it look at the ball, eyes riveted on the exact point of contact. And let it listen for the reassuring sound of a solidly struck ball.

▙● START SLOW; THEN ACCELERATE

The golf swing starts slow, then accelerates. Remind yourself of that before every shot. Don't get it backward. It's a continuous series of lever actions that begin casually and finish compellingly. Many players bolt into the swing, taking the club back abruptly, then float into a downswing that does not gain momentum. To coordinate your body levers, you must start slow, almost lazily for the first twelve inches, and then build speed to finish fast. Not "fast" as in being hurried, but in the regard of gaining pace throughout the swing, no matter what club you are using or how far you want to hit the ball.

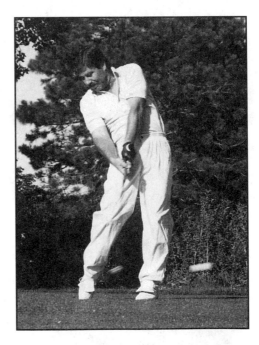

STAY EXTENDED THROUGHOUT SWING

The left arm is the arc-controlling spoke of the swing wheel. Keep it comfortably extended into the backswing. It will bend slightly and quite naturally at the top of the backswing, but it's difficult to reproduce a consistent swing if it's allowed to collapse. The feeling to try for as you unwind into the hitting area is one of unstrained extension of the arms to create a wide sweep of the club, keeping the arms straight as long as possible after impact. This will make it easier to achieve an accelerating rhythm and control and will give you a greater sense of leverage throughout the swing.

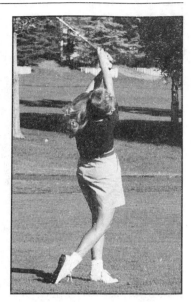

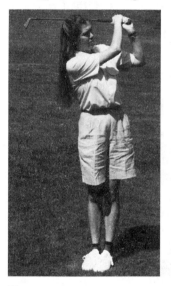

THINK RHYTHM AND TIMING

Tense muscles produce a rigid swing — with nervous shots that are scattered and faulty. The first requisite for a smooth, coordinated swing is to remain at ease. If you concentrate too intensively on the mechanics of the stroke, you can tie yourself into a constraining knot. Create an image of sweeping through the swing. Give each swing a fluid motion with a casual start, then a compelling middle, and an unchained finish. A way to rehearse this is to stand with feet together, then swing the club rhythmically back and forth. Feel the **flow** of the movement. Don't strong-arm the swing. Let it be continuous, pendular-like, without strain.

STAY IN MOTION

Avoid freezing into a static position before the swing, as if posing for a picture. This would produce a start to the swing like a suddenly released spring. Instead, stay in motion. Use a **waggle**. That's a subtle and perpetual animation of your body to keep your muscles from locking into a stiff, pre-swing posture. Try it as a loose-wristed wave of the clubhead along the target line, while at the same time reconfirming your point of aim and making small final settlements of your stance. Experiment also with a **forward press** — a slight move toward the target with the legs, or hips, or hands, just before starting the swing.

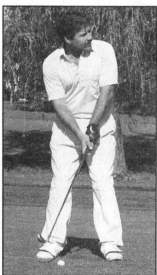

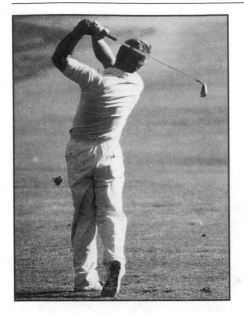

▚• DEVELOP ONE SWING RHYTHM

Every stroke in golf is a variation of a single swing theme. It's a wind and an unwind. The body coils in preparation for the hit, then uncoils with rhythm and increasing momentum. Coil and uncoil. It's a compact maneuver for a short shot, and a free sweep for a drive. But no matter what the distance objective, the basic swing rhythm remains the same. A gradual start, and a flowing finish. It's even true for a putt. So whatever club you pick up, as you practice your swing say "back aaaannnnd throooogh. Learn the timing. Make it a fluid, continuous motion. It'll be a useful attribute for every club and for every shot.

▚• GET TO KNOW ALL CLUBS

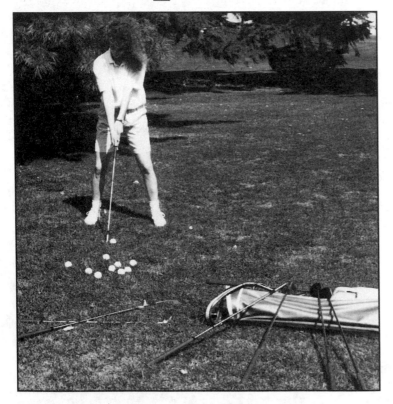

Golf is played by touch. You **sense** the rhythm of the swing, and **feel** the weight of the club. Get to know the difference in the tactile sensation of the clubs by changing weapons often during practice. Recognize the character of each one. Note the typical distance and ball trajectory each produces. You'll automatically start adjusting your stance for each club, and soon develop a catalogue of how the ball behaves with different swing intensities using the same club, or the same swing intensity using different clubs. Eventually your sense of feel will become so refined you can pick up any club blindfolded and know which one it is.

SEEK ADVICE

Inevitably there are times when nothing seems to go right. No matter what you do, your brain does not effectively communicate with your body, and your swing feels like you're a puppet-on-a-string. What to do? Avoid making any sudden or drastic changes. Instead, get a second opinion. Sometimes an observer's eyes will detect things that evade your inside feelings. Maybe you're swinging across the target line, or you're holding your weight on the back foot. Whatever the origin of your woes, another person — your instructor in particular — may be able to discover a mechanical mistake that can easily be rectified and your grief will end.

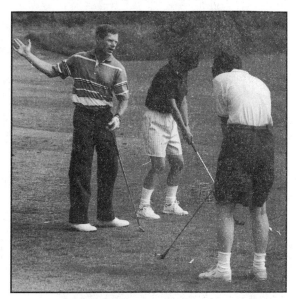

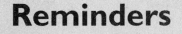

Reminders

1. Grip the club diagonally across the palm of your left hand, but in the fingers of your right hand.

2. Don't exaggerate any aspect of your stance. Be relaxed.

3. Set up with the ball at the bottom of your swing arc.

4. Use a one-piece takeaway to initiate the backswing.

5. Start slowly — gain momentum as the swing progresses.

6. Keep your head steady. Strive for a full swing arc.

7. Give rhythm to every hit. Produce smooth strokes. Flow through every swing.

Problem Solving

Problem	Probable Cause	Possible Solution
Not contacting the ball squarely	Improper position of the ball in setup	Find bottom of swing arc; position ball there
	Body sway during swing	Keep head steady throughout swing
Lifeless ball response	Swing too placid	Gain momentum throughout swing; emphasize follow-through
Tight, jerky swing	Body too tense	Relax grip. Let body be limber, arms loose
	Static starting posture	Stay in motion; use a waggle
	Trying too hard; forcing the swing	Sense the rhythm of the swing; hit with free-flowing motion
Uncoordinated swing	Disjointed takeaway	Start backswing as a unit; arms and shoulders together
Too much wrist in swing	Trying to snap club into ball	Keep wrist action natural, not predominant
Inconsistency in aiming	Improper alignment in setup	Align feet, hips, shoulders parallel with target line

From Tee
To Fairway

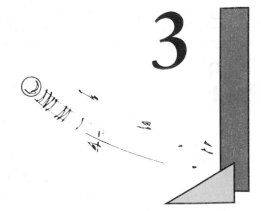

The pursuit of golf is often a compelling quest for power. It's understandable. There's a lot of acreage on a golf course. So it only seems logical to try to get the ball from here to there by hitting it as far as possible. Moreover, human nature being what it is, there's a pure innate pleasure in sending the ball into oblivion. It's emotionally dazzling. And it's dynamic, expressive, lively golf.

Absolute power is absolutely rewarding. To crush the ball on the clubhead and feel the resounding "whack" of the impact, then to watch the ball dissolve into an aspirin-sized missile as it climbs into weightlessness — this is one of the most satisfying moments in sports.

But . . .

An obsession for power can be crippling. It can coerce one into a swing of reckless abandon which decreases the chances for control. It's of no use to drill the ball into long flight if it finishes in a jungle of weeds or admidst a stand of trees. Even the pros rarely swing at full throttle, for the **control** of power is more important than power itself.

And yet, in contrast to this, during the learning stages of golf it's not uncommon to find players cautiously trying to steer the ball straight with a conservative swing, then later trying to hit for distance. In reality it's more economical to first learn to hit hard with a freewheeling swing and then, when tapering the swing off to hit more for control, accuracy becomes remarkably easier to achieve. The moral of this? First learn to hit the ball with power. Turn your swing loose, but within the guidelines of the discussions that follow.

⌊• THE DRIVING SWING

There is no single depository of power. It comes from the whole body. But it is not an act of brawn. It's more a matter of the always influential factors of rhythm and timing. It depends, above all else, on coordination. The north of the body must work with the south, and east with west, all to get the clubhead going at good speed, because the distance the ball will achieve is dependent on how fast the clubhead is traveling at impact.

How to get the clubhead traveling fast? In two basic ways: (1) **linear momentum**, resulting from a subtle shift of weight toward the target, and (2) **rotary momentum**, coming from an uncoiling of the body during the

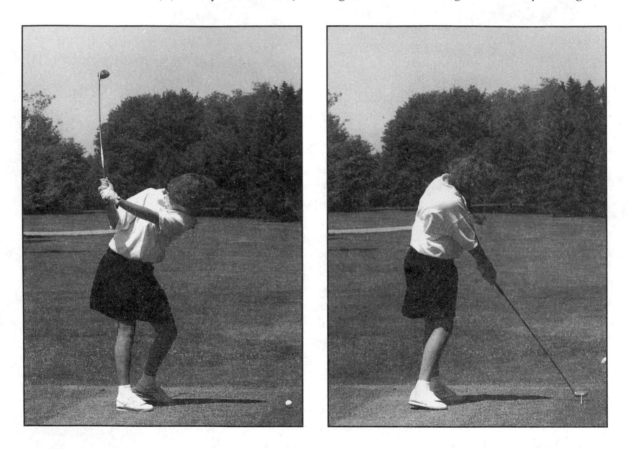

downswing. Both join together in a sequential chain of events that has the following order: (1) with the completion of the windup, the weight transfers from right foot to left, (2) both knees move laterally toward the target, (3) hips turn to open up, and (4) the arms whip the club into the ball.

The end product of these integrated forces is more than the sum of the parts. It's an unrestricted swing of a linear move toward the target, yet without a body sway, and a rotary gyration that utilizes the levers of the body to produce a wide-arc sweep of the clubhead. Never is the swing **forced**. Instead, it emanates from controlled energy. It's a **fluid** motion — muscles in full cooperation with one another. When properly executed, it leaves the hitter with the feedback sensation that the swing was almost effortless rather than a struggle.

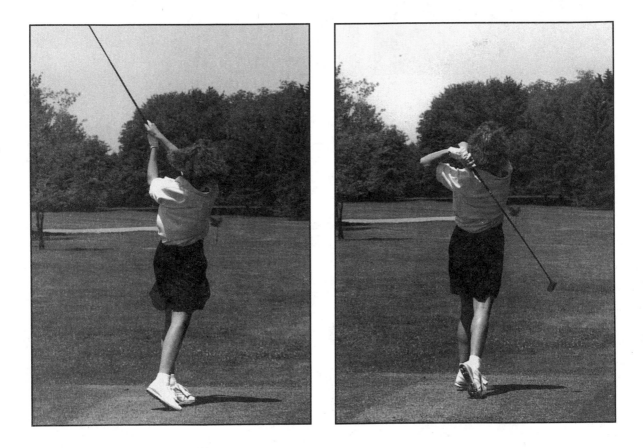

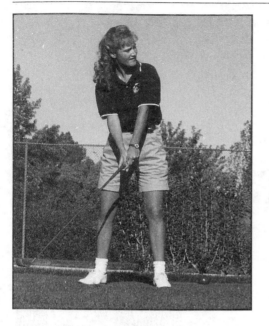

USE LESS MUSCLE FOR MORE DISTANCE

It is often believed that hitting harder comes from swinging harder. So it's common to inadvertently overtry: squeeze the club with a vice-tight grip, firm up the shoulders, speed up the backswing. But the result is a body that's tied up into a constraining knot. Instead, **relax** your body. Consciously untie your muscles. Let yourself go limber — not to where you're unresponsive, but rather relaxed and ready. Stay loose, yet alive and energetic. Slacken your arms, starting with the moment you walk up to the tee. Stay in motion to avoid freezing into a static stance. Then take the club away from the ball leisurely and deliberately to ensure a limber swing.

GET A FULLY EXTENDED ARC

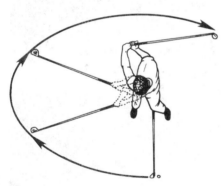

The bigger the arc of the swing, the better the chance of hitting the ball for distance. Increase your swing arc by keeping your left arm fully extended into the completed backswing. Don't lock your elbow, or force your arm into a splint-like rigidity, but do stretch out for a wide sweeping arc. At the top of the swing, feel like you're "reaching for the sky" with both arms. Start the downswing only after you've felt your hands high above your shoulders. Think of your left arm as the radius of this big arc, and the downswing will have the natural effect of centrifugal force to speed the clubhead assertively into the ball.

WIND UP WITH UPPER BODY

There's torque in your torso, ready to be released like a spring. Wind up this physical spring with a slow start back, taking the club around your spine with a spiral of your upper body. Stay extended with your arms to promote a wide-arc swing. Let your hips be pulled around by the shoulders as you wind up. The further and tighter you can wind up your lower

body against the resistance of
your lower half, the more you'll
feel a great sense of multiplying
power and energy. It may seem
you've corkscrewed your skeleton
into the configuration of a question mark, but you have coiled
yourself for a reflexive strike at
the helpless ball.

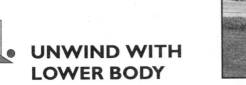

UNWIND WITH LOWER BODY

At the completion of the windup the torsion between the two
halves of your body will be so great that the muscles demand
immediate release. So send the club on an accelerating journey.
Release your physical spring to discharge the energy from the
ground upward: left heel replants solidly, both knees move laterally toward the target and hips simultaneously rebound from
their twist, the backbone uncoils, and the shoulders and arms
catapult the club into the ball. It's a whip-like continuous sequence of lever actions that start slowly, then finish explosively.
Remember to **allow** this to happen rather than **forcing** it. Sense a
freedom in your swing with loose, lively arms.

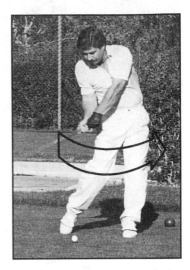

ACCELERATE THROUGH THE BALL

It's a physical law. A clubhead that is accelerating at
impact will impart more force to the ball than if the clubhead has the same speed but no acceleration. Stay tena-
ciously active through the hitting zone. Make the clubhead gather momentum so it comes into the ball while
still gaining speed. Instead of hitting **at** the ball, think of
hitting **through** it and a couple of feet beyond. Take a lesson from karate. To break a board with the bare hand it's
essential to imagine a contact point on the **other side** of
the board and then swing for **that** point — not the board
itself. So imagine the ball isn't there. Hit beyond it.

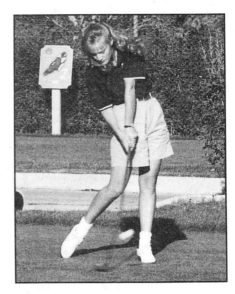

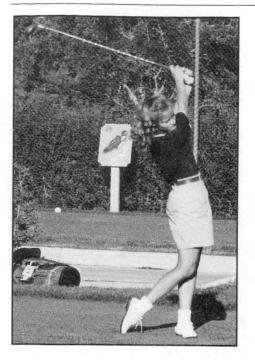

FINISH THE SWING

If the clubhead is lazy at impact, the ball will feel heavy, like a hunk of lead. But if you've accelerated **through** impact, the ball will feel like it has virtually no weight and will spring into noticeably livelier flight. It even **sounds** different — a higher pitched "thwack" instead of a dull "thunk." When all goes well, your clubhead will carry into a long follow-through. You feel **unwound.** Hold your finish position for a second to check where the clubhead is. It should have wheeled up over your shoulders to end by pointing more or less toward the ground, providing evidence that you had a beyond-the-ball acceleration in your swing.

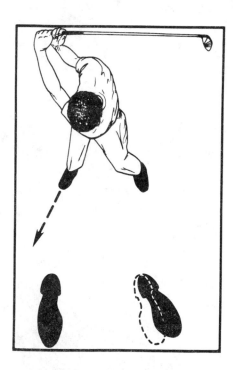

ADJUST THE STANCE

Standard opinion is that the right foot, in a power swing, should be aligned ninety degrees to the target. But if you're having trouble achieving a full coil in the windup, such foot placement may be acting as an anatomical brake to restrict your backswing. Compensate by turning your right foot away from the target, opening it only far enough to allow you to get the club, at the end of the backswing, pointing toward the target. On the other side, make sure your left foot is turned outward enough to allow your hips to rotate and clear the way for your arms to swing cleanly past your body. Experiment on both sides to where your swing feels unrestricted.

EMPHASIZE A WEIGHT TRANSFER

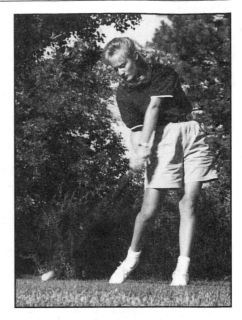

Optimal power will not be generated without a weight transfer. It's common, when overhitting, to hold the weight on the right foot during the downswing. Thus linear momentum is lost, and the hitter has only the rotary component to deliver the power. Push off the **inside** of your right foot to start the downswing, and this will encourage both knees to move toward the target, along with your weight. Do that **before** your upper body begins to unwind. It's a tricky maneuver, but it will give more whip to your swing. Keep both knees flexed through impact, and remember that even though you're striving for a free-wheeling swing, everything must still be under control.

Reminders

1. Stay loose, limber, alive before the swing. Keep tension out of your arms.

2. Strive for a wide arc in the swing. Use your left arm as the radius of this arc.

3. At the top of your backswing, feel like you're reaching for the sky.

4. Wind up by coiling the upper body, but unwind by sequentially unwinding from the lower body.

5. Gain linear momentum by shifting the weight toward the target in the foreswing.

6. Accelerate through the ball and a couple of feet beyond.

7. Let the club finish on a path up over your shoulders, coming to rest pointing downward.

8. Generate a feeling of expressive energy release through the swing.

Problem Solving

Problem	Probable Cause	Possible Solution
Lack of control of swing	Overswinging; trying to hit too hard	Hit at only ninety percent of maximum effort
Not getting full coil in backswing	Foot placement restricting backswing	Rotate right foot outward to allow full coil
Contact of ball is not solid	Tensed-up swing	Relax whole self, especially arms, before address
Lack of weight transfer	Weight stays on right foot during downswing	Push off inside of right foot to start downswing
Still lacking power	Too confined a swing arc	Keep left arm extended as radius of wide arc
	Starting downswing with hands and arms	Start downswing with lateral knee movement and unwind hips
	Clubhead quitting	Accelerate through and beyond ball

From Fairway To Green

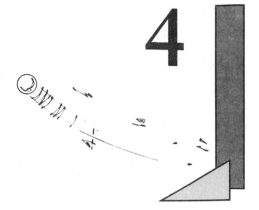

In golf lingo, they call it "getting up and down." It means getting the ball up onto the putting green and down into the cup — with the least strokes. It's decisive golf. To score well requires performing this part of the game with a good show of dexterity and accurate aiming.

This chapter is about getting the ball up — from the fairway to the green. It describes **approach shots,** which are those hit with the intent of having the ball finish on the putting surface.

It's **touch** golf. Approach shots ask for a deftness of skill to **finesse** the ball to its appointed destination. They verify that golf is a game of seeing and feeling. To strike an accurate approach shot, you must first see the distance the ball should travel, visualizing the scene with the eye of a surveyor. Then you must feel the alertness of your muscles as you prepare them for a swing of the proper magnitude. Miss an approach shot and it's costly to your score, but lift one adroitly into perfect flight and a gentle finish on the green, and suddenly your psyche comes alive.

There are two basic, but related, approach shots. The **chip shot** is hit from close in to the green. From further out, the stroke takes on the characteristics of a **pitch shot.** The trajectory of each and the optimal roll after landing depend on the nature of the swing and the club used.

Approach shots are a great equalizer. They can compensate for a mediocre drive, or rescue the ball from a poor lie, or make putting an easier task. Acquiring an aptitude for these shots is, therefore, the quickest way to lower scores. It could be argued that they are the logical starting place for learning golf. So if your lessons have begun with a focus on approach shots, they have been aimed at the very core of the game.

THE CHIP SHOT

From near the green, when there are no hazards between the ball and the hole, the appropriate ploy is to hit a chip shot. It's a short, crisp strike of the ball. The objective is to lift it over the longer grass around the green to land on the putting surface and amble up to the hole. There's no attempt to give the ball backspin to retard its roll, as in a pitch shot. Rather, the ball should find its distance by roll as well as by flight.

The shot does not have any of the conscious body rotation that is used for a full swing. All that's needed is an unrushed, even-paced pendular motion with minimal wrist action. It's a firm, controlled **sweep** at the ball where the club just brushes the grass to spank the ball on its way. In fact, the swing more closely resembles a putting stroke than a full shot. In

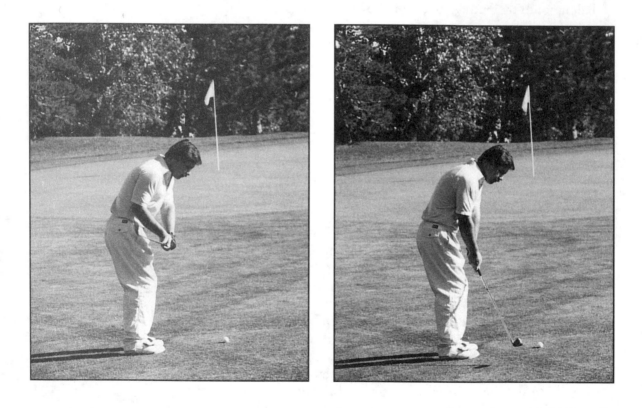

further fact, some players **think** of the chip as a long putt hit with an iron instead of a putter.

Watch the pros hit chip shots, and you may get confused. Some use a pronounced wrist action; others swing with stiff wrists. In general it's much more reliable to keep the wrists steady, though not locked, for the whole swing. It's predominately an arm action rather than a wrist or shoulder motion.

The length of the shot is determined primarily by the length of the backswing. Too short a backswing can lead to stabbing at the ball with a stilted stroke. Too long a backswing can encourage a slowing of the club as it approaches the ball.

There's nothing complicated about a chip shot. It starts with a careful reading of the needed distance; next a few rehearsal swings to prime the muscles; then a proper setup, and a neat, packaged, resolute swing. The biggest thing is to keep from being surprised at how easy it was.

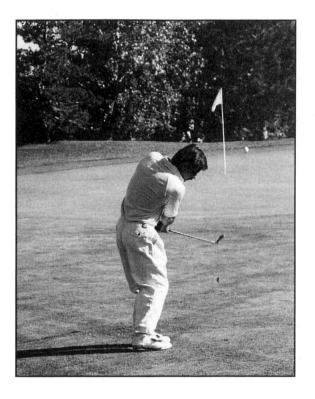
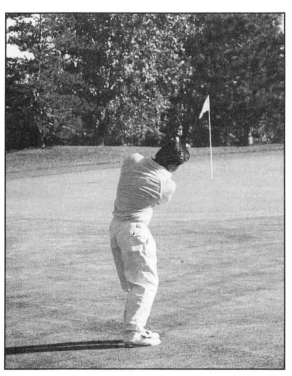

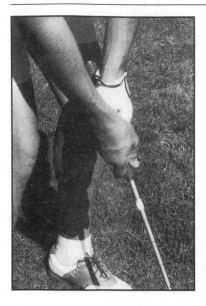

1. TRY THESE SETUP ADJUSTMENTS

Choke Down for Control

On short shots there's more need for touch. If you move your grip down for a chip shot, you'll use less shaft and therefore be closer to your work. This will provide for better control and a more delicate touch. Choke the club at least halfway down on the grip, and choke down to the same extent for all your chipping clubs to standardize their feel in your hands.

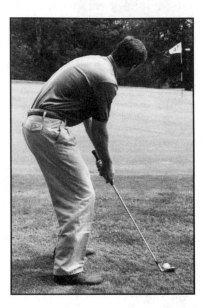

Set Up Closer; Open the Stance

Stand relatively close to the ball, without crowding it or feeling constrained. This will facilitate a more direct swing path, and a better chance for square contact. Then open the stance. The closer setup could fix your left side into a static block of a free-swinging motion. But the open stance allows for a smooth swipe at the ball and an unrestricted follow-through.

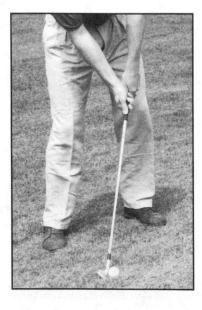

Set Hands Ahead of Clubhead

Address the ball with your hands forward, ahead of the clubhead and toward the target. This will keep you from hitting the turf before (or instead of) the ball. It also encourages a swing that keeps your wrists steady and moving on-line to the target. Lay more of your weight onto your left foot at address, and keep it there throughout the swing to facilitate a smooth, pendular motion.

TAKE A CONVINCING SWING

Here's a real key to a successful chip shot: it should be an unfaltering swing — **smooth** and **deliberate** — a positive, firm stroke. A common tendency is to decelerate the clubhead as it approaches the ball, as if the guilty golfer is saying "I'm not sure about this," and the attempt becomes a gentle nudge instead of a convincing stroke. So the biggest obstacle might be psychological. A chip shot is an uncomplicated task. There's no body rotation to worry about and little if any weight transfer. Talk yourself into it. Get a sensory awareness of the club. Then, instead of a cement-arm swing, take an unhurried, fluid, determined stroke, and command the ball to seek its target.

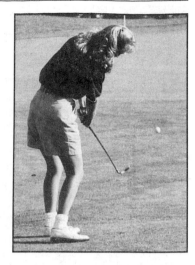

AIM FOR THE GREEN

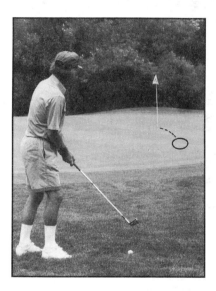

On short shots, whenever you can land the ball on the green, make that your objective. Start analyzing the lie as you walk up to the ball. Visualize where you want the ball to land. See the shot having two parts: one being flight, the second being the roll on the putting surface. Judge how the ball will behave on its roll. Have all this planned even before addressing the ball. Choose a club that will provide the proper flight and sufficient roll. Then pick an aim point on the green for your target. Focus on that aim point, take some practice swings to cue your muscles, set up properly, reconfirm your aim point, and hit a smooth, positive stroke.

A COMMON ERROR

The biggest blunder on a short chip is scooping at the ball in the mistaken belief it must be dredged from its lie. So the left hand could collapse as the right hand dominates the stroke (as shown). Strive instead for steady wrists. Help your cause by keeping a consistent grip pressure throughout the swing. Then think of hitting **through** the ball instead of under it. Say "throooough" as you swing into the ball.

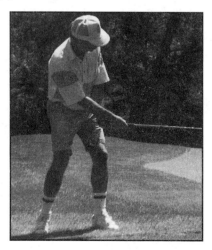

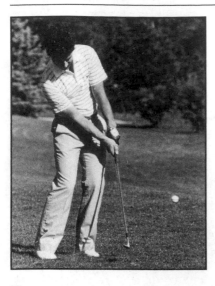

⌐● USE YOUR HANDS AS A UNIT

There's little wrist action to a chip shot. It's similar to a putt, in which the wrists are held steady, and the left hand is the guide. Practice this feeling by chipping with your left hand only. Be firm in this one-handed swing. Then lay your right hand on the club and swing with the sensation it's moving **with** the left instead of over and around it. Finish with the clubhead still on the target line.

⌐● CHOOSE THE RIGHT CLUB

Deciding which club to use for a chip shot is critical. Learn this judgement by first chipping to one spot with the same club until you're consistent. Next, use the same aim point with other clubs and observe the difference in roll. Adjust the aim point to compensate for the roll each club produces. Then chip from different distances, and with different clubs. Soon you'll know which club gives the best results for given distances.

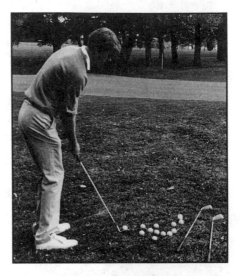

Reminders

1. Set up relatively close to the ball, then open the stance.
2. Choke down on the club; set hands ahead of clubhead.
3. When practical, aim to land the ball on the green.
4. Prime the distance of the shot by the length of the backswing.
5. Use the arms to control the shot, with minimal body rotation.
6. Keep the wrists steady throughout the swing.
7. Sweep the club forward, just brushing it through the grass.
8. Take a smooth, positive, convincing strike at the ball.

Problem Solving

Problem	Probable Cause	Possible Solution
Inconsistent flight and roll	Improper club selection	Learn club selection by practicing with different clubs
No life to shot	Decelerating clubhead at impact	Take a fluid, confident swing; emphasize on-target follow-through
Hitting turf behind ball	Jabbing at ball	Stay unhurried; focus on rhythm of swing
Erratic contact; unpredictable flight	Scooping at ball	Keep wrists firm; hit through the ball, not under it
Pulling shot to left	Right hand overpowers left	Let left hand lead the swing, both hands working as a unit
Poor control of shot	Holding club at end	Choke down halfway on handle
	Standing too far from ball	Move closer to ball; open the stance

⬛◦ THE PITCH SHOT

The situations that ask for a pitch shot can vary markedly. There can be a need to loft the ball forty yards over a massive sand trap to an elevated green or a one-hundred yard straightaway shot to a flat, unobstructed green. In all instances the objective is to park the ball on the putting surface, but the conditions can be so diverse that the pitch shot, it is often said, is the most troublesome stroke in golf. It requires less than a full swing, yet it's not the neat little parcel of a chip shot. It needs body rotation but not the full coil of a drive. Most crucial of all, it demands a sensitivity for swinging the club with just the right measure of strength for the needed distance.

But the rewards are great. When you can hit pitch shots with confidence, the club becomes an extension of your arms and the ball your

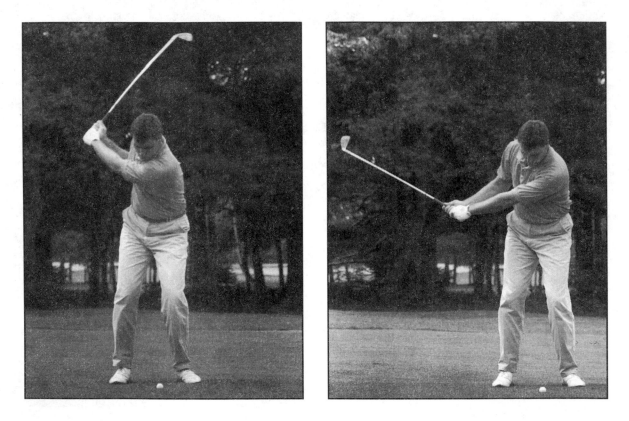

servant. Best of all, your acquired talent for pitching the ball from its various settings onto the green is an aptitude that lifts your entire game — to pitch well is to play well.

From near the green the shot is similar to a chip — slightly open stance, hands laid ahead of the club at address, and a swing of steady wrists. As the distance from the green increases, the technique begins more and more to resemble a full swing.

Several factors determine the success of a pitch shot. One is an accelerating clubhead at impact. Another is staying firm on the feet for the whole swing, with the weight mostly on the left foot at impact. Another is a backswing of proper length for the distance the ball is to be hit — the swing merely becomes a little longer with any increase in distance needed. But a sense of rhythm and timing and gathering momentum must govern all shots. The **quality** of the swing does not change just because the club in the hands does. Instead the club and desired distance will determine the **quantity** of the swing and resulting compulsion given to the ball.

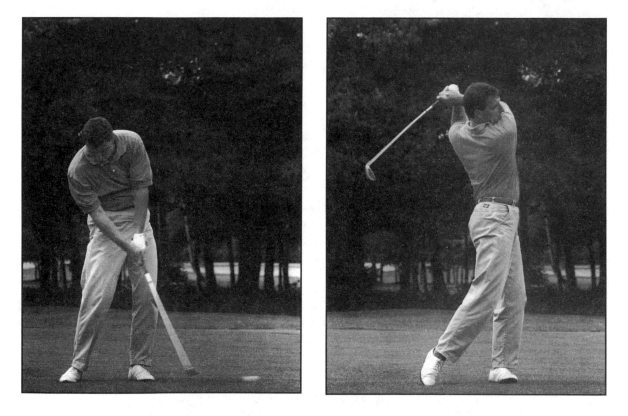

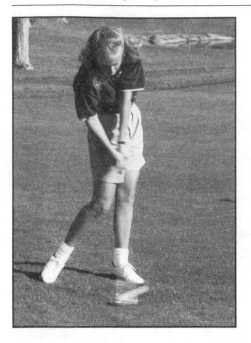

▌. ACCELERATION IS VITAL

A decelerating clubhead in a pitch shot is crippling. It produces a listless ball. The usual cause is too long a backswing, followed by a hesitant downswing. It's often a mental thing — an overenthusiastic windup that changes in midswing to an indecisive slap of the ball. Instead, convince yourself that the clubhead needs acceleration. Talk yourself into a positive reference, ready to take an affirmative stroke. Swing with authority, whether it be for a hundred-yard whack with a 3-iron or a forty-yard loft with a 9-iron. Then watch with pleasure as the ball kicks responsively off your club, hangs weightlessly in the air, and alights smartly on your aim point.

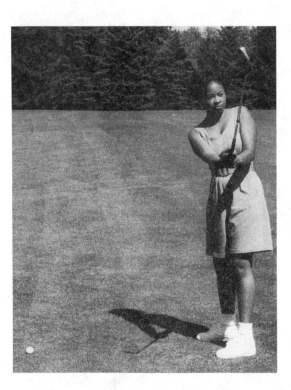

▌. FIRST DECIDE;
▌. THEN REHEARSE

Prepare for a pitch shot by first surveying the land carefully. What is the lay of the terrain? Are there hazards? Where should the ball be aimed, and what is its behavior likely to be after landing? Use all your resources of logic, and fix your decisions in your mind before addressing the ball. Choose the club that will provide the right loft and distance. Take a rehearsal setup and two or three practice swings. Send a message to the muscles, telling them exactly how active they should be. Then step up to the ball confidently, deliberately. Stay loose, alive, limber. Simply let your body act out your swing decisions.

PRACTICE FROM DIFFERENT DISTANCES

There is no typical pitch shot. Each situation on the course is unique. Distance is always a variable and the major judgment factor in planning the shot. Consequently, learning to control distance is a prime requisite. Head for the practice range or to a local park where you can set out targets at, say, twenty, thirty, and fifty yards. Choose one club, preferably a 7-iron. Try for the shortest target first, then work up to the longest, and finally mix up the shots, all with the same club. This will sensitize your feel for that club. Then try the same scenario with a different club. Note especially how the length of the backswing is closely related to the length of the shot.

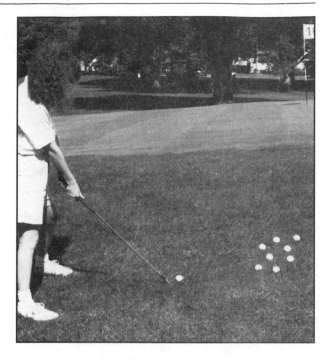

PRACTICE FROM DIFFERENT LIES

Prepare for variable sittings of the ball by tossing a handful of balls randomly onto uneven terrain. As you practice from their different lies, see the importance of a solid stance, durable wrists, and a firm strike of the ball. There's a tendency to let the left arm get lazy and bend during the pitching swing, so emphasize it especially now by keeping it extended through the full arc. Keep your heels down for each shot and make the action of your right arm similar to throwing a softball underhand. Sweep the clubhead forward so that it just clips the grass. Don't take a divot. Hit the ball, not the turf.

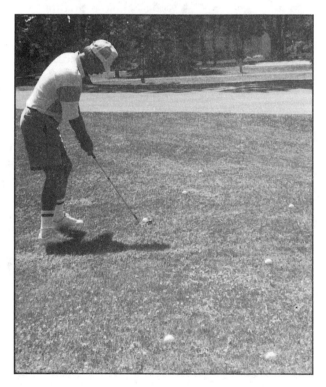

LEARN HOW TO GET HEIGHT WHEN YOU NEED IT

During any round of golf, there will be situations where you'll need to hit the ball high and bring it to a halt soon after landing. Most typically, this will be when you must cross a sand trap to get to a green. Not only must the ball be lofted, but it must also have backspin to "sit down" on the green instead of bounding off the back side. Confronted with this ticklish circumstance, golfers often get weak knees.

There's a tendency to tighten up for this shot, so unlock your arms. Your swing must now be expressly unconstrained — free and flowing.

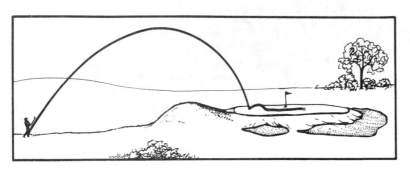

Clear your psyche with your best self-talk for the right frame of mind.

Take out a sand wedge. It's the most lofted club, and having the weight set low on the blade gives it the advantage of being able to more easily kick the ball into the air. Don't have a sand wedge? Use a pitching wedge. Don't have that either? A 9-iron will need to do, at least until you add a wedge to your set of clubs.

Set up so the ball is at the **bottom of your swing arc**. Since you'll often be on uneven ground, test this with practice swings to see where the bottom of your swing arc is relative to your stance.

Unlock your wrists. You need to give the ball emphatic backspin with this shot to park it near the landing spot. Firm wrists tend to nullify the loft of the clubhead, thereby reducing the height and backspin of the ball. The same is true if your hands are laid forward at address. Align your hands more directly with the ball. Take a relatively slow backswing to emphasize the importance of a smooth, unfaltering stroke. Make an especially authoritative swat of the ball with your right hand.

USE A PITCH AND RUN WHEN PRACTICAL

There are other situations where the territory between the ball and the flagstick is unobstructed and relatively flat. The ball will not need height, so the choice in this case could be a **pitch and run** (sometimes called a "bump and run"). In contrast to a high lofted shot, the objective of a pitch and run is to have the ball collect most of its distance by bouncing and rolling. In general it's a safer shot, less susceptible to mistakes, and is an especially logical play when the green is firm and would therefore nullify the braking power of a lofted backspinning ball.

The pre-shot planning is that of a chip shot. Judge two parts: (1) the pitch, or, flight of the ball, and (2) the run, or its expected bounce and roll. If possible, find an aim point that is smooth and flat so the ball will not rebound unpredictably after landing.

Which club to use? Try a 7-iron. It has about the right loft for this shot. If it's a short distance you need, choke well down on the club, almost to the steel. For all pitch and run shots, **lay your hands decidedly forward**, toward the target, as you set up. Put stability into your wrists, and determine to keep them secure for the swing, not allowing them to hinge very much in the backswing.

Make a clean hit of the ball. Spank it with solid impact, culling it cleanly off the grass without picking up any turf. Let the clubhead follow into the intended line of flight, as if you're pointing with the club to tell the ball, "go there!" Then be ready to acknowledge the plaudits of your playing partners as your ball rambles neatly up to the flagstick.

Reminders

1. Survey the needed distance carefully. Find an appropriate landing point for the ball.

2. Take several practice swings to prime your muscles for the correct backswing length and downswing intensity.

3. Apply the same relative power to all shots, varying only the length of the swing.

4. Be extra cautious of keeping the left arm extended through the entire arc of the swing.

5. Accelerate the clubhead into the ball.

6. When lofting the ball, unlock the wrists and set up so the ball is at the bottom of the swing arc.

7. For a pitch and run, set hands well forward and keep steady wrists throughout the swing.

Problem Solving

Problem	Probable Cause	Possible Solution
Undependable distance of shot	Needed distance not judged correctly	Use trees, flagstick, etc., to help give perspective for distance
	Swing was not primed	Take several practice swings before setup
Hitting too short	Clubhead decelerating at impact	Keep club actively moving through impact
Inaccurate shots	Improper setup	Double-check aim relative to setup
	Left arm collapses in swing	Keep left arm straight for full arc of swing
	Unsteady body	Stay firm on feet for entire swing; heels down
Inconsistency on lofted shots	Choppy stroke	Take a smooth, unhurried swing
Not enough backspin on lofted shots	Wrists too far forward at setup or impact	Keep hands aligned with ball at address; unlock wrists
Ball flies too high and too short on pitch and run	Swing too much of a regular pitching stroke	Set hands forward at address; keep them forward throughout swing

On The Green

5

There's a timeworn saying; "Drive for show and putt for dough." It exemplifies the importance of skill on the green. Hit the ball a long way off the tee and it's impressive, but it's the work of the putter that produces low scores. Miss a point of aim by ten yards or more on a drive and it usually doesn't matter. The ball is still out there, having collected the objective of distance. But miss a putt by a mere inch and the score jumps by an extra stroke. Even a drive that finds the rough still leaves one with a chance to recover with the next shot. But a missed putt is a dead loss, without reconciliation.

Consider this: the par assigned to any given hole is the score an accomplished player is expected to achieve on that hole. To originally establish par, two strokes are automatically allocated, on every hole, to putting. With eighteen holes, that's thirty-six total putts for the round. Par on most golf courses is seventy-two. So the golfer who would play a hypothetically classical round by scoring the assigned par on every hole would have used half the strokes in putting.

On the green — it's where the game gets tedious. To putt well requires control of mind and physique. It calls for an acute eye to judge with the precision of a surveyor how the ball will probably roll. And then, with the mental blueprint in place, there must be a keen sense of touch to send the ball, with proper pace, on its designated route. All the power from the tee and the sureness of the approach shot now converge on this: a gentle tap of the ball to complete its journey to this final puncture in the green. It is, literally, a game within a game.

◣. THE PUTTING STROKE

To describe a certain putting techniques is vulnerable to question when watching a Sunday afternoon telecast of a golf tournament and there, in full witness on the screen, are a wide range of putting styles. Yet within this assortment of forms there are certain common features.

Much of the success of the stroke is in setting up, carefully checking — double checking — the planned route of the putt. Nothing is rushed. The ball is not hit until there's a resolute decision about its projected pathway nor until there's a correct setup alignment for sending the ball on that path.

The stroke itself is a skill of virtually no body movement. It has the character of a grandfather-clock pendulum motion. Imagine a fulcrum in

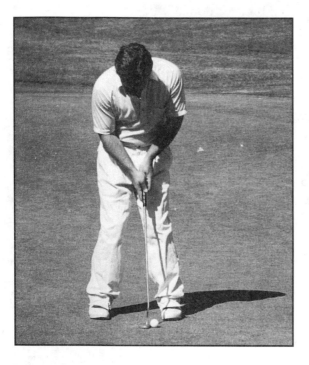
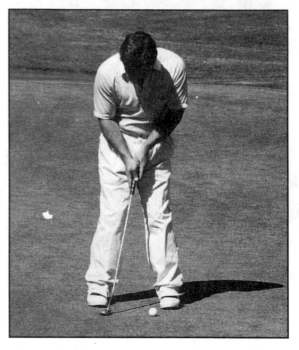

the neck, with the shoulders and arms assuming full responsibility for swinging the club. No wrist action is needed, for that would oscillate the club too abruptly up and down and make the stroke choppy. Steadiness is the key — steadiness in stance, in body, in head, in wrists. Like all other strokes, the putting swing has its own rhythm, its own pace, and a commitment to firmly bringing the clubhead into and through the ball, without forcing the stroke. In fact, the putter seems almost to swing naturally of its own weight.

As is true for approach shots, the length of the putt is predicated on the length of the backswing. The pace of the backswing determines the pace of the foreswing. It's a metronome stroke, back and through, with a flow of rhythm that makes for a well-timed hit. When everything is in sync, the biggest problem is to remain humble as putt after putt drops neatly into the hole.

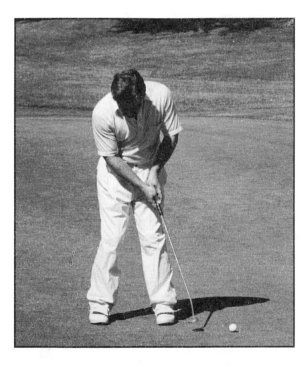 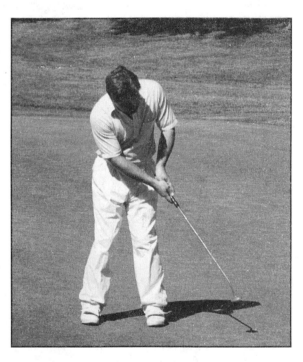

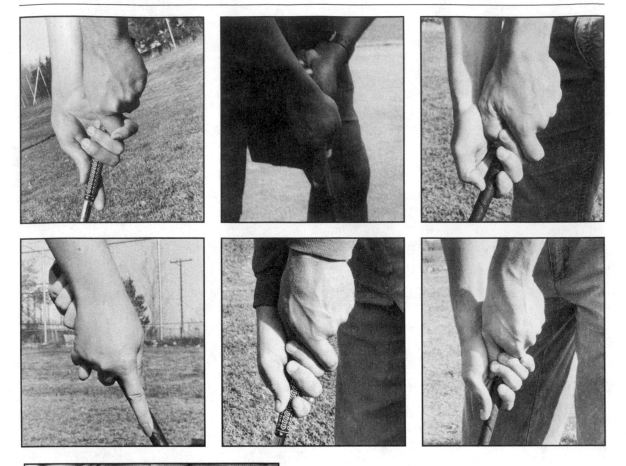

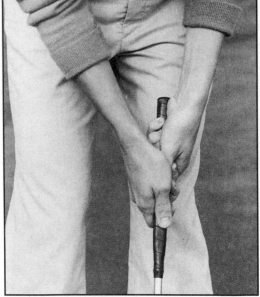

GET A COMFORTABLE GRIP

Find ten golfers and you might see ten different ways of holding the putter. It's because putting depends on **feel,** so it's vital to have a grip that's **comfortable.** Logic is to have the palms face each other and aligned with the putter head — palm of right hand toward the target line. This should give the feeling the back of the left hand will guide and the right hand will "push" the putter head along the target line and squarely into the ball. Keep grip pressure moderate and assign "touch" for the stroke to the forefingers of the right hand.

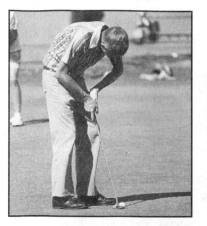
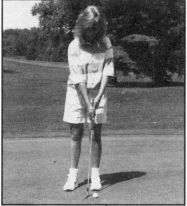
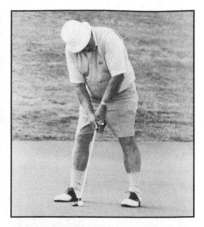
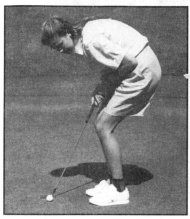
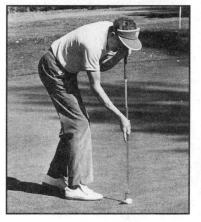
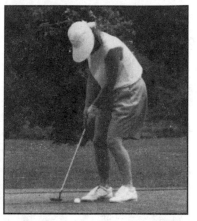

⌊• FIND YOUR BEST POSTURE

There are also incredibly diverse ways of setting up. What is best? Consider this: putting needs no lower body movement, so almost any posture will do if it provides **stability** to hold your head absolutely still for the stroke. Keep your weight solidly balanced, perhaps slightly toward the left heel, and hold it steady for the stroke. Set your feet about shoulder-width apart. Bend over enough to let your arms hang freely away from your body. Have your eyes directly over the ball or over the target line slightly behind the ball.

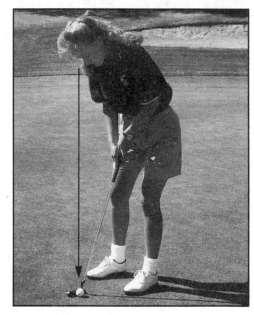

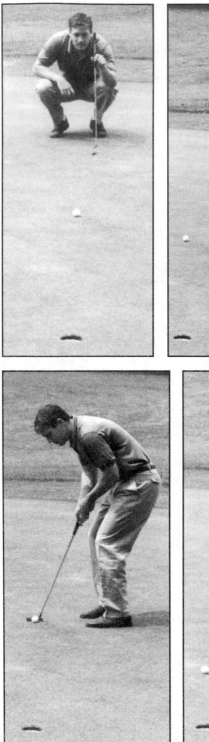

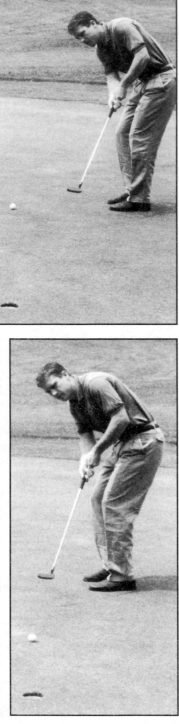

⌊• DEVELOP A PRE-SHOT ROUTINE

It makes good sense to have a consistent pre-shot routine to properly prepare for the putt. Start by scanning the green as you approach it, noting the overall contour of the surface. Get different viewing angles to form a general idea of how you think the ball will behave on its roll. Make your final judgment by looking down the anticipated target line from behind the ball, surveying the terrain from both a crouch and while standing.

Having decided on the line for the putt, move up next to the ball for a few practice swings. Take your normal stance, and make the practice swings true preludes of the putt you want to hit. Prime your muscles. Tell them exactly what you want them to do. Bring your confidence up to where you're **sure** the ball will find its mark.

Hold the sensation of the proper swing in your muscle memory, step up to the ball, and adjust your stance until you're satisfied you're in proper alignment. Double check the target line. Double check it again.

All is in readiness. No thoughts now of the mechanics of the swing. Think only of rhythm and a solid hit, then let your body act out the swing you just rehearsed. Watch the ball drop into the cup and tell your playing companions how easy it was.

KEEP THE PUTTER UPRIGHT

Keep the putter plumline straight at address. If, in your stance, you sight the ball from slightly behind, it makes it easy to tilt the club back and increase the pretense for striking the ball on the bottom of the blade. Or, if your weight is too predominately on your left foot, you could unknowingly be tilting the club forward, with a likelihood the ball will be punched into the turf. Set up with the putter blade **flat** on the ground, and avoid any forward or backward tilt of the hands. That way you'll have a more consistent swing, and you'll give the ball true end-over-end roll instead of a dribble.

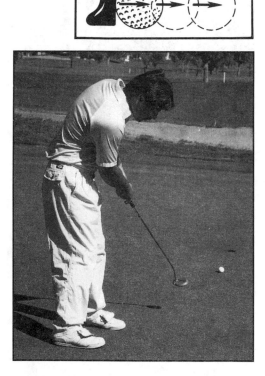

KEEP ELBOW BEND CONSISTENT

Since putting is a pendular motion, the arms and shoulders must cooperate as a single unit. This means the bend of the elbows should be a constant for the stroke, especially the left elbow. If it extends during the backswing, the putter will be "dragged" awkwardly into the foreswing as the elbow reinstates its bend. Instead, hold the left elbow steady with the same crook it had at address. And don't let the right elbow stray too far from your side, where it will throw the clubhead off the target line and close the putter face. Keeping the palm of your right hand facing the target will help with swing stability.

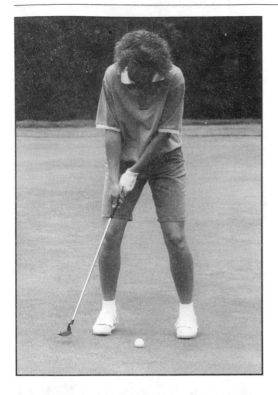

SWING WITH PENDULAR RHYTHM

Rhythm!! It's an important ingredient in every golf swing. It's **crucial** in putting. Often a tendency is to punch at the ball, like a boxer's jab, and the ball responds erratically. Give rhythm to your putting swing. It can have a slow or fast pace, so long as it has rhythm. Activate it with the backswing, which should have the same pace as the foreswing. Press your left thumb firmly on the shaft to serve as a fulcrum — the pivot point — of the pendulum swing. Still feeling tight? Take the putter back further than you had been and swing more easily into the ball. It will smooth your motion and soothe your nerves.

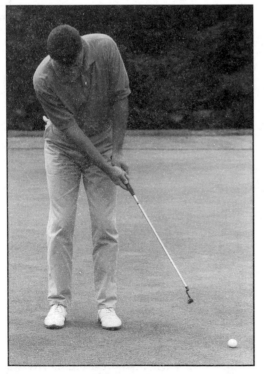

KEEP A QUIET HEAD AND BODY

No need for any body motion in putting. You could have your head in a vise, and it should have no effect on your stroke. But some players will shift their head forward along with their swing, as if to urge the ball into its roll. Another tendency is to lift the left shoulder in the foreswing, thus lifting the putter to plunk the top of the ball. All this makes for a stilted, ungainly swing. Think of your neck as the pivotal part of your swing. Keep your head steady, your body quiet. Make your arms and shoulders a unit. Let your hands regulate the momentum of the swing.

ON THE PRACTICE GREEN

Three-Ball Drill

Practice greens are easy to find. Use them often. Here's a suggested drill. Set out three rows of balls, three in each row. Putt the first one, giving full attention to the sense of touch needed for the distance. Then putt the next two with eyes closed. Observe the result and give your muscles information about any needed adjustments. Do the same for the remaining two rows of balls. The objective is to give **feel** to the swing.

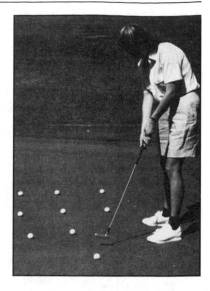

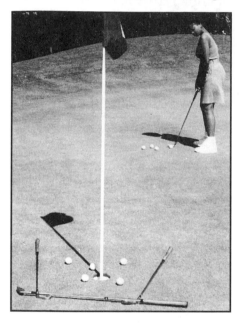

Get Long Putts Close

On long putts a common philosophy is to lag the ball up close to the hole so it can be one-putted from there. The concept is that it's safer and more consistent to try for a larger target than the cup itself. So imagine the hole is a large bucket with a two-foot radius. The objective is to get the ball within this target. Practice this tactic by laying clubs around the hole to provide a goal.

Build Your Confidence

Be sure to also practice shorter putts. On the course, a missed short putt is a bruise to one's psyche. Build confidence for these short ones by spreading a circle of balls around the hole. Hit them one at a time, moving around the circle. Not only will you develop sureness in your swing, but as a bonus, you'll get to read the pitch of the green from lots of different angles for the same hole.

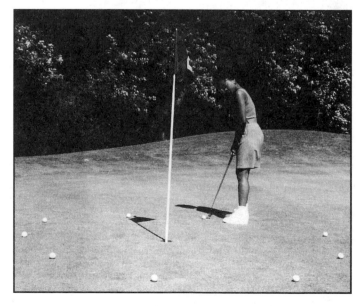

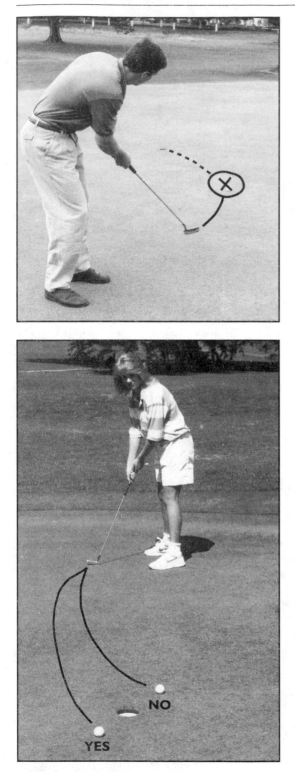

FIND A SPOT FOR BREAKING PUTTS

Knowing how to putt is half the story. Knowing where to putt is the other half. Every green is different. Sometimes it seems they're built on a mountainside. Whenever you expect a big curve in the path of the putt, try a technique used by experienced bowlers. They "spot-bowl," aiming for a spot on the alley rather than the more distant pins. The theory is it's easier, and psychologically more comfortable, to hit a closer target. Try this tactic. First visualize the anticipated route of the putt. Superimpose in on the green, actually seeing the line. Then pick a spot near where the putt will begin its curve and aim the ball for that target.

NEVER PUTT SHORT

Always give the putt enough mileage. Leave a putt short and even if it's right on target, it can't drop. The moral: Always hit with enough length to have the ball go slightly past the cup if it misses. That way you'll hole the ball when the aim is true. It's especially critical for breaking putts. The tendency is to be conservative in estimating the degree of break, and consequently to send the ball curving short of the cup. Aim for the high side of the hole, and give the ball enough fuel to make it at least that far so it can fall in neatly, or literally drop in through the "back door."

Chapter 5 On The Green 49

DOUBLE BREAKING GREEN IS TWO PUTTS IN ONE

So here you are, on the green but miles from the cup, and the landscape in front of you shows that the putt will break twice, in opposite directions. The ball will start out on a slope and curve away from it, but then change course to bend the other way as it sweeps around another, opposite slant of the green. It's a double whammy — a roller coaster ride that tests the judgment of your telescopic eye.

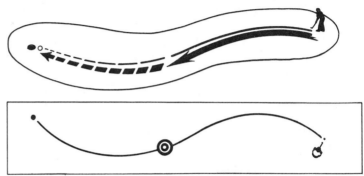

Divide the putt into two parts. First visualize the expected curve on the near slope, then isolate the far slope as a separate putt. Remember that the ball will be traveling considerably faster on the first incline, and this will reduce its curve. But its bend will magnify greatly as it slows down on the second pitch. Keep this in mind as you analyze both hillsides. Now identify a point along the route where the second break will begin to take effect. Make this your target. It will give you a definite and positive point of aim to hit for instead of swatting the ball with only an amorphous idea of what path it might take. Be sure to give the ball a vigorous start, then watch it snake its way up to a parking place near the cup.

Reminders

1. Have a consistent pre-shot routine for reading the green, then practicing the swing, and setting up to putt.

2. Find a comfortable grip, with hands aligned parallel to the putter blade, palms facing each other.

3. Assume a setup which provides stability for a steady body and quiet head throughout the stroke.

4. Maintain a constant bend in the left elbow for the stroke.

5. Use little or no body movement for the swing.

6. Swing with a pendular, rhythmical, even pace.

7. Guide the club along the target line with the left hand, and push it with the right.

Problem Solving

Problem	Probable Cause	Possible Solution
Inconsistency in results	Failure to analyze green prior to putt	Develop a routine for reading green, swing rehearsal, and setup
Erratic length of putts	Forcing the putter head forward in swing	Swing with same pace on all putts; vary distance by varying length of backswing
Problems of direction	Pulling head forward or lifting shoulder with foreswing	Hold head and body steady for swing; pivot arms around neck as fulcrum
	Punching at ball	Take slower backswing, longer follow-through
	Pulling club off target line	Keep clubhead square to line through impact
	Using wrists for swing	Keep wrists steady; keep club on-line past contact point
Unpredictable response of ball	Putter tilted forward or backward at contact	Keep putter vertical, with blade flat at address
	Too stiff a backswing	Slacken arms; hit through the ball

Saving Strokes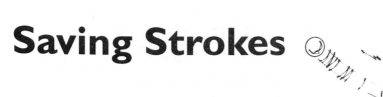

The first golf courses, laid out during the Middle Ages along the eastern seacoast of Scotland, were grass-tufted sand. The courses were **sand**. Any incidental growth of grass was considered a hazard. Time changes things. On today's finely manicured grass courses, it's sand that is the hazard.

There are sand traps guarding almost every green. No golfer can continually escape them. Sooner or later one of them will swallow up a smartly lofted approach shot that would otherwise have bounded from just off the green to within one-putt distance. In the midst of green pastures the ball will have found a wasteland.

If sand traps aren't enough, there are other perils to test a golfer's resolve. Drives curve off the fairway to plummet into the rough, or into a vale of trees, or both. And then the game is instantly reduced to one simple task: getting out of the hazard in one shot. It's loosely referred to as "scrambling," and the shot you hit to get back into play is called a recovery shot. The best recovery is a shot that leaves you with a good clean unobstructed lie for the next stroke. So even if you hit a bad shot, you can repair the mistake and go on to produce a satisfying score on the hole. As you walk off the green, no one will ask how, but rather how **many**. A par will be a par, no matter how much scrambling you needed to get it.

Many players lose their cool when they leave the fairway, and therefore they further compound their original mistake. But here's where you can cut your losses and save strokes. This chapter describes recovery shots, starting with how to pull out of a sand trap. We'll see that the sand trap isn't the most exquisitely tortuous hazard most golfers believe it to be.

┗● THE SAND SHOT

With few exceptions, the sand trap will be below the level of the putting surface. So the ball must be popped into the air to clear the lip of the trap and land on the grass. The proper club for the task is a sand wedge or, in its absence because of economics, a 9-iron.

Getting out of the trap requires an "explosion" shot, so called because the ball is propelled into flight by a blast of sand resulting from the impact of the clubhead. So the objective is — and here's the psychological barrier — to hit the **sand** behind the ball; **not** the ball. If the intent were to try to swipe the ball directly off the sand, any inaccuracy in contact could easily thunk the ball deeper into the sand, or send it flying across to the opposite side of the green.

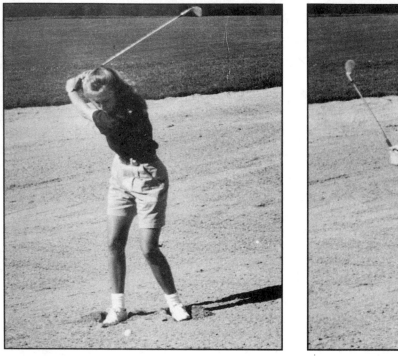
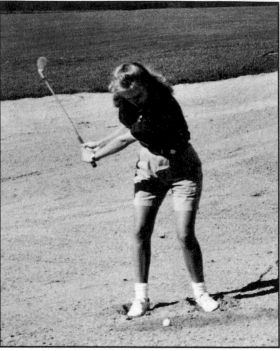

Common flaws in the swing are: (1) to scoop at the ball in the mistaken belief it must be shoveled into the air, or (2) to chop the club downward thinking it must be forcefully muscled into and through the sand. In truth the swing should have much the characteristics of a pitch shot, although experienced players will send the club into the sand at a slightly steeper angle than for a shot hit off the fairway. An important criterion is to keep the hands moving convincingly through the hitting zone to compensate for the resistance of the sand. The swing must have determination, without being forced. It needs a solid kick into the beach and a follow-through of high finish to guarantee that the clubhead does not quit as it meets the sand. And the swing must maintain the basic essentials of any golf stroke: rhythm and timing.

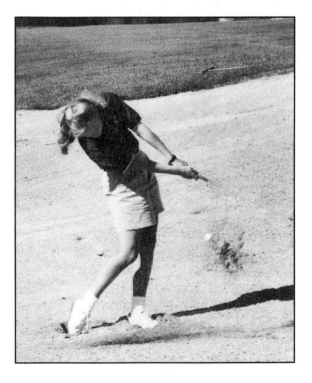
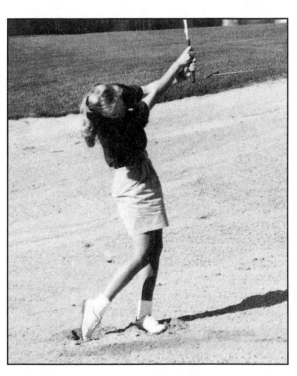

OPEN BOTH CLUB AND BODY

A common technique among experienced golfers is to prepare for the sand shot by opening both their setup and the clubface, then swinging on-line relative to their opened stance. This facilitates the knifing of the club-head through the sand, and the ball surprisingly responds with a proper

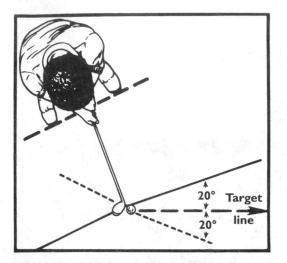

flight path. Aim your shoulders, hips, and stance to the left of the target, but lay the clubface off to the right. Keep both opened angles similar. If you set up, say, twenty degrees left, lay the clubface open twenty degrees to the right of the target. Have the ball slightly forward of center, but aligned in relation to your opened stance and anticipated swing path.

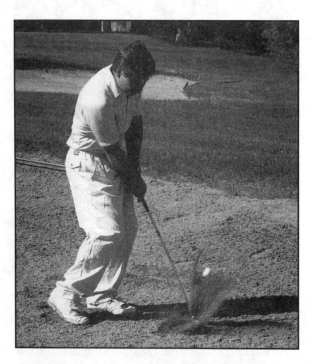

USE THE SAND

Take a shoulder-wide stance, then scrunch your feet well in to the sand, especially if it's soft or sugary. Twist well in until the sand is above the soles of your shoes so you have a firm foundation against the instability of the sand. This will set you down lower than normal, so you may need to compensate by shortening up on the grip an inch or so. Then **forget any ball fixation.** Don't address the ball. Mentally exclude it from the picture. Address the **spot in the sand** you want to hit, and swing directly for that spot. Have faith the club will do the work by exploding the ball into the air as you contact the sand.

⌊• FINISH THE SHOT

Take plenty of time setting up, focusing intently on the spot you want to hit. Then be deliberate, almost slow-motion, to start the swing. Take a backswing that's comparable in length to what you would take for a chip shot of twice the distance you need at the moment. The biggest objective is to make sure you don't quit with your hands, especially not letting your right hand overpower the left in the downswing, for that would close the clubface at impact. Use a normal swing arc, without attempting to spade into the sand. But hit with conviction. Propel the clubhead through the sand to finish high. Tell yourself before you swing to **finish the shot.**

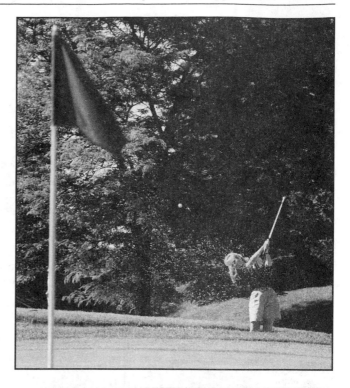

⌊• FIND A PRACTICE BUNKER

A major reason for any neurotic fear of sand traps is from never having practiced in them. Find a practice trap, then try this gimmick. First make your own lie by building a little mound, about half an inch high. Place a ball on top, and swing so your club takes the sand from under the ball. This will help you to get the feeling of hitting something other than the ball. Next plop the ball down on level sand, and trace a rectangle in the sand surrounding the ball. Make your aim point the back of the rectangle, and then try to remove the entire rectangle of sand from under the ball as your swing. Soon the sand will no longer be a threat.

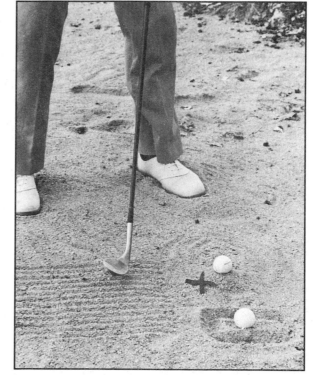

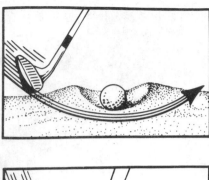

⌊. DIFFERENCES IN SAND

The Fried Egg

A lofted shot descends vertically and — splack! It leaves a depression that looks like a fried egg. Important now is to make sure you cut enough sand from under the ball. Don't aim too high on the mound; the club will take off the lip and then contact the ball directly. Keep the clubface squared for-this one.

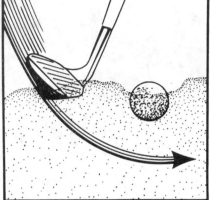

Buried Lie

Square the clubface so it will knife into the sand rather than sliding through. Lift the club more sharply in the backswing, using more wrist, for a steeper angle of attack. Swing more downward without overdoing it. Be emphatic. The club might actually stay in the sand as the ball explodes out.

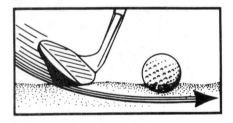

Wet Sand

Here the tendency is for the club to bounce off the sand and ricochet into the ball. To compensate, use a pitching wedge, then with a firm swing try to skim the ball off the sand instead of kicking the club into it. You might try an open clubface. Allow for extra roll of the ball. It's an easier shot than it seems.

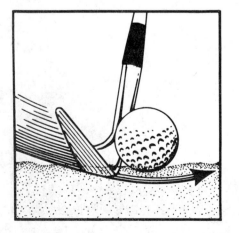

Hard Sand

If the ball is sitting up high on compact sand, consider hitting a regular chip shot. Just take a firm swing to pick the ball off cleanly. Be sure to keep your head steady, and allow for distance just as in a normal chip. If there's no lip on the front edge of the bunker, you might even try putting the ball out.

⌐● FROM THE ROUGH

A predominant golfing hazard is the rough, which borders most fairways. It's an ecosystem that can provide unlimited hiding places for the ball. Eventually every golfer gets into it. How, then, to get out?

If the ball has a reasonably unobtrusive lie in dry, light grass, it can be played normally. But if the ball has found its way into long or lush grass, the way to hit it out effectively is with a more descending blow using a lofted club. A regular, sweeping swing would catch too much grass before arriving at the ball. Bring the club back with an early hinge of the wrists to produce a steeper arc. Lead the downswing with your hands. Hit especially hard with your right hand — use a "throwing" action. Keep your eyes riveted on the back of the ball. Open the clubface before swinging, because the rough will generally twist it closed as it grabs hold of the club. Don't be afraid to use a well-lofted wood if it's distance you need from the shot.

Otherwise you could decide to "punch" the ball out with a more rigid swing. If so, be sure to lay your hands distinctly forward at address and determine to keep them ahead of the clubhead through impact.

Remember that grass growing away from the target will offer more resistance, while growth toward the target gives less resistance and the ball will probably fly a greater distance.

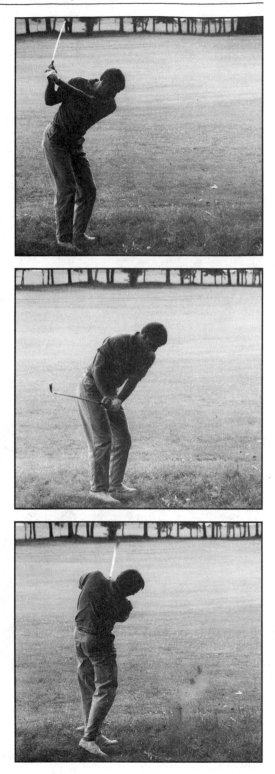

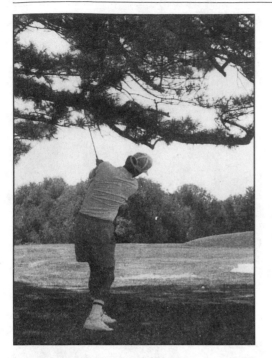

PUNCH THE BALL UNDER BRANCHES

Say you're within pitching distance of the green, but overhanging tree limbs prevent you from hitting a normal iron shot. Keep the ball under the limbs by playing a punch shot. Choose a club with less loft. Set up so the ball is in the center of your stance. Lay your hands well forward. Give more weight to your left foot and keep it there during the swing to prevent body sway. Do not take your hands higher than shoulder level in the backswing. As you swing through the ball, keep the back of your left hand definitely facing the target. For this shot you really need to stroke the ball firmly, without any conscious wrist action.

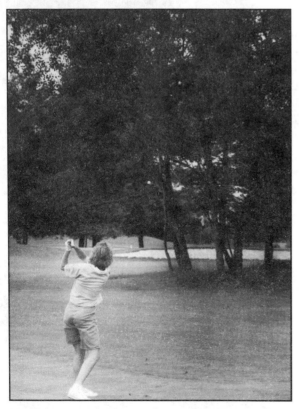

RELEASE WRISTS TO CLEAR TREES

Hitting over trees isn't nearly as difficult as is often believed. The stroke is played with much of the character of a bunker shot. Open your stance slightly, and also the clubface. This will automatically increase the loft of the club, although diminishing its distance potential. Position the ball up front, near the left foot, but not so far forward that you would risk drilling the club into the turf before hitting the ball. Add a bit more wrist hinge to an otherwise normal backswing, then release your wrists fully as you come into the ball. If it's a short shot, fifty yards or less, use a sand wedge. For greater distance try a less lofted club.

⌐• UNEVEN LIES

Uphill lie

When confronted with a lie on an uphill slope, set weight into hill, flexing your uphill leg to maintain stability. Otherwise, try to simulate a normal stance. Have the ball well forward. Bring the club back low and swing **up** the slope for the hit. Release good wrist action on this shot.

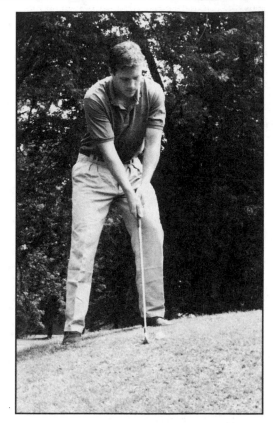

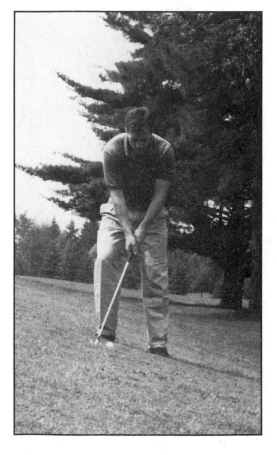

Downhill lie

Settle weight mostly on your rear foot, and hold it there, to maintain balance on the swing for a downhill lie. Set hands ahead of ball. Use a quick pickup of the club in the backswing, and chase the clubhead down the slope and through the ball. No "scooping." Use a sufficiently lofted club to get the ball airborne.

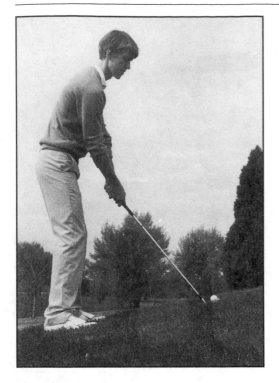

Ball above feet

Stand more erect than usual when the ball is above your feet. Set weight toward toes. You may want to choke the club enough to keep your arms extended. Swing in a compact arc, more around your body, to sweep the ball off the hill. The ball tends to come out to the left, so compensate by aiming to right of target.

Ball below feet

Hunker down for this one, bending at knees and, mostly, the waist. Have weight on your heels and stand close to the ball. Swing more upright, which will restrict body coil, so use predominately your arms and hands. The common flaw is raising up during the swing, so keep your head absolutely still. Aim left, because ball will want to fly right.

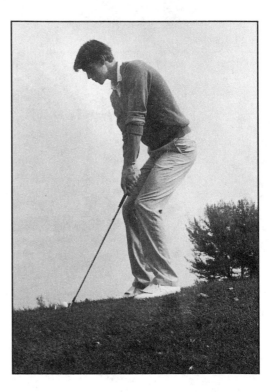

Reminders

1. For a sand shot, open both stance and clubface equally.

2. Pick spot in sand, behind ball, as aim point for bunker shot. Focus intently on spot, not on ball.

3. Swing firmly, staying active through sand. Finish shot.

4. From the rough, make swing more upright; use more wrist.

5. To stay under tree limbs, hit punch shot with hands forward and wrists firm.

6. To send ball over top of trees, release wrists fully.

7. On uneven lies, align body with slope; swing clubhead more parallel with slope, maintaining steady head throughout.

8. For hilly lies, guard against unusual body sway during swing.

Problem Solving

Problem	Probable Cause	Possible Solution
Ball flies too far from bunker shot	Hitting ball instead of sand	Find aim spot in sand; forget the ball; swing for aim spot
Ball never gets out of sand	Scooping at ball	Make swing more like pitch shot
	Chopping club downward	Hit firmly through sand; finish shot
Club "quits" in sand	Swing too passive	Keep hands active through sand
Sluggish ball response out of rough	Too much "sweep" in swing	Lift club early in backswing; use more wrists for hit
Ball will not stay down under tree limbs	Swing too much like normal pitch shot	Lay hands and weight forward; hit firmly with steady wrists
Ball does not get high enough to clear trees	Swing too stiff	Set ball forward; hit like long bunker shot; use active wrists.
Trouble with uneven lies	Improper setup	Set up to allow as normal swing as possible

Cures For Faulty Shots

There was a research physicist who, in a rather whimsical mood, obtained data relative to how exacting human muscular movement could be, then multiplied the error factor by the length of a driver, added the parameters of physics that determine effective clubhead-ball impact, and came to the conclusion that a human being was not capable of generating the accuracy of movement necessary to drive a golf ball into straight flight. A lot of players might nod in condescending agreement.

A few zillion things, it seems, can go wrong in the few seconds it takes to crank up one's body and slash the club into the ball. And when the ball does not find the target, it can reduce the golfer to a quivering despair or frustration. Hitting an errant shot is not only excruciating in itself, but it also leaves one in the unfortunate predicament of a resulting poor lie, and this may increase the probability of yet another erratic shot. Hit a disastrous shot in tennis, by contrast, and the next point starts anew. But deliver a lousy shot in golf and it infects the next stroke as well.

Fortunately, the protocol of a deviant golf shot is based on two general principles:

1. Every mistake has a cause, therefore;

2. Knowing the cause, a cure can be prescribed.

To eliminate a faulty shot means first determining the cause and then reorganizing the swing accordingly. Thus, no mistake in golf need be a constant. The remedy is simple — find the cause, then effect the cure. After all, the physicist who concluded that a ball cannot be hit straight also "proved" that a bumblebee cannot fly because its wings are too small for its body mass. But bumblebees can fly.

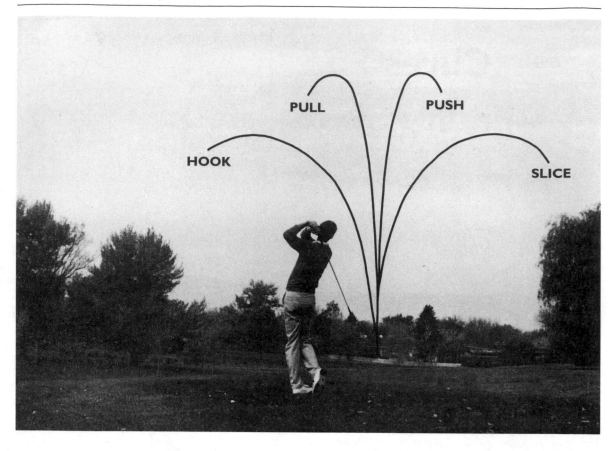

PULL PUSH

HOOK

SLICE

▌. FOUR COMMON FLIGHT DEVIATIONS

There are basically four kinds of errant flight that can result from improper alignment of the clubhead at impact. A **push** and a **pull** will stray from the target line, right or left, but essentially in a straight path, whereas a **hook** and a **slice** will arc in a continuous curve away from the target.

What causes the errors? The ball tells the truth. It goes where it **must** go, according to physical law. It takes its flight pattern from instructions given to it at the moment of impact by two determining factors: (1) the direction the clubhead was traveling, and (2) the angle of the clubface. Once airborne, the ball reveals both factors. It has no other choice. So it's easy to know what the behavior of the clubhead was during the microsecond it was in contact with the ball. Less obvious, but still discernible, is what went on at the other end of the club — with the golfer's swing — to cause the incorrect pathway or clubface angle.

▐• SLICING AND HOOKING

If the ball takes a curving detour in its flight, it tells that the club was not, at impact, squared off at ninety degrees to the swing path of the clubhead. If the club arrives at the ball with an open face (turned outward, to the right of the swing path), the ball will have no choice but to bend into a slice. If the club-face is closed at impact (turned to the left of the swing path), the ball will acquire a hook. A slice is by far more common. It's a golfer's nightmare. A persistent slice can become so devastating as to ruin one's enjoyment of the game. Yet there may be a simple remedy.

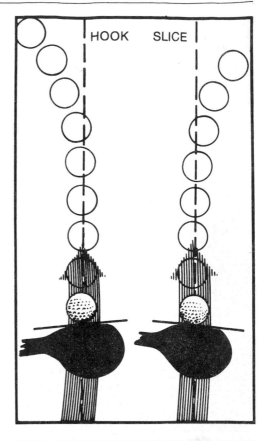

▐• A POTENTIAL INSTANT CURE

If the ball generally starts its journey on the target path but then, as it gains altitude, veers off into a slice or hook, the solution might be a simple realignment of the grip. If it's a slice, the clubface is open at impact because the hands have not returned it to the squared-up position it had at address. Rotate your grip to the right — clockwise on the handle — so your hands can more readily pull the clubface around during the swing. Gradually shift your grip until the ball assumes its proper flight. If it's a hook, do the opposite — rotate your grip to the left. You've just saved a twenty-dollar golf lesson.

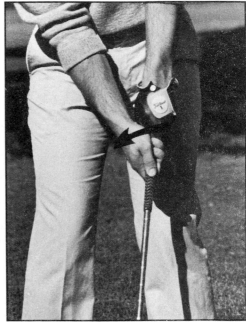

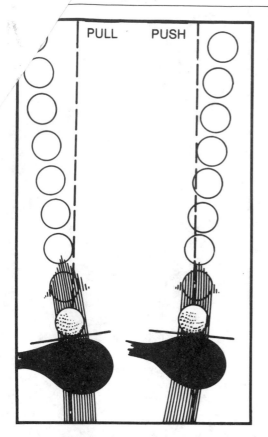

PUSHING AND PULLING

If by rotating your grip you have straightened out a slice or hook, but the ball still flies off target, you have either a push or a pull. A push is a ball that, though straight in flight, is sent to the right of the target. A pull also goes straight, but to the left of the target. A pull, surprisingly, is often the aftereffect of a slice that was corrected by a realigned grip. A push often follows a repaired hook. When the club-face has been properly squared off relative to the swing-path of the clubhead, any deviant ball flight now comes from an error in the **direction** of the swing path. You're ready for stage two of the renovation.

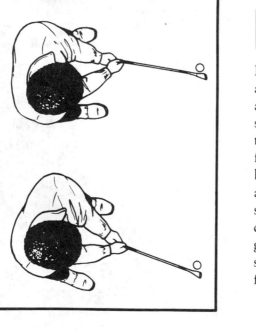

TWO SOLUTIONS

First check your setup. If you're not squarely aligned at address, your swing path will reflect your misalignment. That's actually good news, for your swing is correct. It's simply misdirected because of the lopsided setup. Square up your shoulders, hips, feet to the target line. If that does not bring you back on target, take note of the position of the ball at address. Playing the ball too far back in the stance can cause a push because it's hit while the club is still approaching along the inside of the target line. A pull can occur from a too-late-in-the-swing contact, fostered by a ball positioned too far forward in the stance.

1. IF YOU'RE STILL SLICING

It is generally estimated that about eighty percent of the people who play golf are afflicted to some degree with slicing. It can be like a persistent cold that won't go away. For the majority, rotating the grip and/or squaring the setup should dramatically reduce the problem. However, if you have made these adjustments and are still plagued by a slice, try the following:

◉ Set the club more into the fingers of your left hand (instead of nesting it back in the palm). This will keep your left wrist from being too firm and blocking the effort of your right hand to square up the club at impact.

◉ Hold the club more lightly at address, especially with the right hand, and maintain an easier grip throughout the swing. A subconscious tightening of the grip, especially the right hand, will keep the clubface open.

◉ Make sure you are not actually opening the clubface at setup. Keep it squared to the target line.

◉ Keep your wrists steady in the early part of the backswing. Emphasize a one-piece takeaway — a unit turn of your body under a steady head — and this will bring the club into the backswing correctly to the inside of the target line. Use less hinge in the wrists for the whole swing.

◉ Slow the backswing and avoid rushing the transition from backswing to downswing. If you spin your body dramatically to the left at the start of the downswing it will pull the club across the target line.

◉ Be sure you are not "throwing" the club from the top of the backswing with your hands to start the downswing. This will force the clubhead ahead of the unwinding of the shoulders and will draw it inside the target line. Instead, start the downswing with the legs and hips.

◉ Swing for less distance. Don't try to overpower the ball, since this can produce a delayed squaring of the clubhead and/or a "falling" of the weight away from the ball.

◉ Pull your right shoulder back, away from the target line at address, especially if you had been compensating for a slice by addressing the ball with a deliberately open stance.

◉ Sense that your arms fully extend, during the downswing, to reach out to contact the ball.

AN OVERALL CHECKLIST

The source of a faulty shot is sometimes difficult to identify. It could be the result of several simultaneous mistakes. The following is a checklist of factors that could potentially contribute to each deviant flight.

If the fault is a: **The potential cause could be:**

Slice	Hook	Push	Pull	
X			X	Grip rotated too far to right
	X	X		Grip rotated too far to left
X			X	Stance too open (misaligned left)
	X	X		Stance too closed (misaligned right)
X	X		X	Ball too far forward in stance
X	X	X		Ball too far back in stance
X			X	Setting up too close to ball
	X			Setting up too far away from ball
X			X	Weight on left foot at address
X			X	Tension at address; into swing
X			X	Rushed swing
			X	Stiff rear leg in swing
	X			Uncontrolled, exaggerated windup
	X		X	Right hand overpowering left on downswing
X				Weight on heels at contact
	X	X		Poor lower body rotation on downswing
	X	X	X	Pulling club inside flight path on backswing
X	X		X	Trying to hit too hard
X			X	Delayed weight transfer in downswing
	X		X	Insufficient shoulder turn in windup
X				Falling back on heels during downswing
	X	X		Swing path in-to-out across target line
X			X	Swing path out-to-in across target line

ON THE COURSE

Sometimes, in the midst of a round of play, you'll suddenly be struck with a persistent flaw, usually an uncontrollable slice. You'll wonder if you brought enough golf balls along. How to save the day? Slow down. Often, slicing occurs in mid-round when you subconsciously start trying to hit harder. It can manifest in a "whirling" windup and a resultant slashing at the ball. Instead, make a conscious effort to be deliberate, especially on the takeaway. Also, the tension of a close match can coerce an abbreviated shoulder turn. Relax your arms. Coil slowly, completely, into the backswing. Then lead the downswing with the lower body so the club releases by a natural effect of centrifugal force.

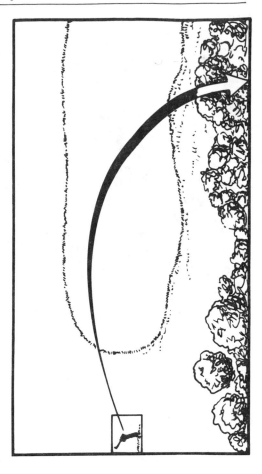

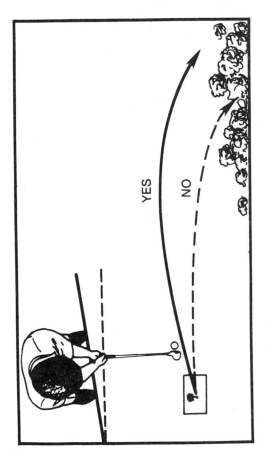

ADJUST TO THE FLIGHT

A moderate rightward curve in ball flight is called a **fade**. It's not as dramatic, or devastating, as a slice. If you have a natural fade, or you have straightened out a slice to where it's now a fade, consider leaving well enough alone. Simply allow for it when you play. Aim down the left side of the fairway by setting up slightly left, and let the ball fade back into the middle. The opposite of a fade is a **draw**. It's a modest leftward curve. If you naturally do that, not to worry. Many pro golfers try to draw the ball intentionally, since it seems to produce longer flight and more roll. In either case, fade or draw, just allow for it.

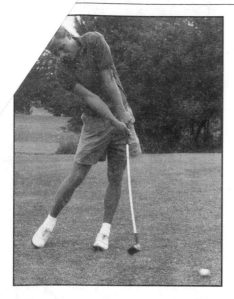

THREE OTHER MIS-HITS

Shanking

When hit off the heel of the club the ball is shanked and heads for the wilderness. The usual cause is moving too far forward, out and over the ball, for impact. It could also be from starting the downswing with the hands, like fly-casting. Correct the flaws with a steady head, and more body rotation to pull the club through the downswing. Also try setting up with weight more toward the heels. Be sure to stay the proper distance from ball in setup.

Topping

If hit with the bottom of the clubface, the ball is topped and never gets airborne. The arc of the swing was too high, usually from rising up on the toes or possibly also from pulling the upper body away from the ball. Both can happen when trying to kill the ball. Cure either case with a fixed axis of rotation around your neck. Stress a long, slow backswing. No rushing. Be sure to shift weight toward the target for the downswing.

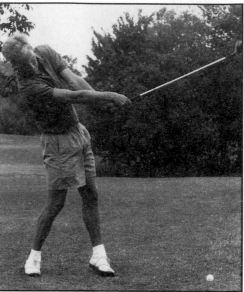

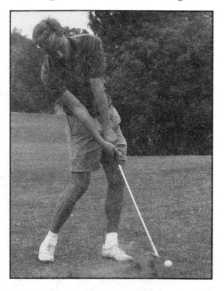

Fat shots

It means hitting the ground behind the ball. One cause: throwing the clubhead ahead of the hands in the downswing. A related cause: weight falling too much onto right foot in backswing and keeping it there for downswing. Antidote for both: keep head in same place for whole swing, and lead the downswing with the left side, club trailing. It helps to set up with weight on inside of right foot, left foot turned more outward.

Getting Better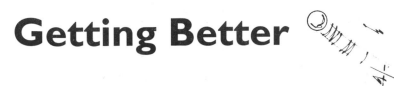

W hat does it take to get better at this game? Skill. Coordination. Desire. Mental discipline. An analytical mind. All these, and more. But there is one important factor that is often short-changed: **practice**. It's the final architect of talent. By law of the human nervous system, no one gets better by accident. The only way to master repeatable skills is by rehearsal.

Sometimes it's a struggle to go from one stage of skill acquisition to the next. Because the game requires precision in execution, progress can seem so slow as to be discouraging. Besides, practice is mundane compared to playing. There's less exhilaration, fewer rewards for doing well, and no penalty for errant shots. But the results of such diligence will eventually show. Any golfers who want to chop a stroke off their score here, another there, the value of practice is foretold. Learning to get good may not be as much fun, but having learned to be good is great fun.

Most important, practice allows one to cultivate an ability to play the game with increased tactile sensation — by **feel**. It's a time when you can freely experiment, thereby opening your mind to sense and learn from the inside information coming from your own muscles, tendons, and joints. By listening to the messages of biofeedback coming through your nervous system, you can literally get inside your muscles to monitor their activity and more effectively control their movements. As a result, you'll become less mechanical, more crafty. Then you'll go to the course armed with not only improved skill, but also an enlivened neural alertness which makes for spirited play.

●. REALISTIC PRACTICE

Knowing **how** to practice is as important as doing so. Quality is more rewarding than quantity, and thought is as influential as effort. Thus any practice session, to offer the greatest returns, should be realistic. It should attend to the overall skills that are needed for the actual game. Accordingly, the following might be considered as guidelines:

- During practice, it's common to hit shot after shot with the same club; yet, on the golf course you rarely use the same club for two consecutive shots.

- During practice it's common to hit shots in punctual succession, but on the course there is more of a time lapse between shots.

- During practice it's common to try mostly for maximum distance. On the course, accuracy and control of distance are more important, and the optimal distance changes for each shot.

- During practice the ball is usually hit from a tee, or at least from a level, unobstructed lie. On the course you often must hit from an angled lie, or from the rough, or out of sand, or around an obstacle.

A well-rounded practice session will include attention to the **total** game, without overlooking such often neglected aspects as the pitch and run, short chip shots, and various recovery shots. Rehearsing a medley of different strokes will make practice more interesting, and give reason to do well.

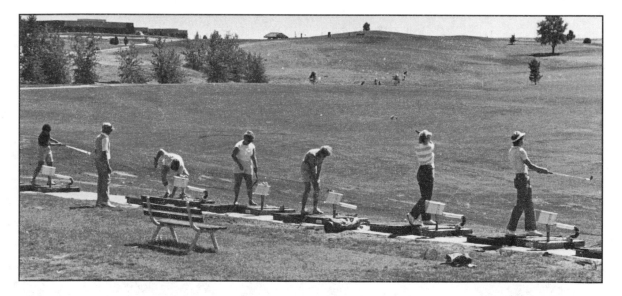

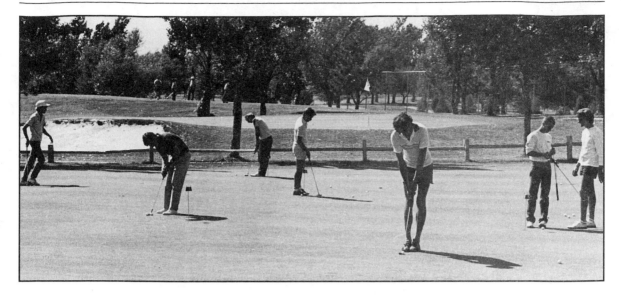

▌. A PROGRESSIVE SESSION

Ordinarily, when people want practice time, they will be off to a driving range. And therein they get a subliminal suggestion.... a "driving" range? So they commonly pull a driver out of the bag and devote their time exclusively to trying to reach the furthest marker.

We all have limited time to practice, so when we do, it should be with a purpose. At a "practice" range, instead of attending only to how far into oblivion the ball can be hit, the major objectives are to:

◉ Be willing to **practice**, which means trying to improve in all phases of the game, not just in driving.

◉ Rehearse the things that will **actually happen** on the course.

◉ Make the session **enjoyable**.

To these ends, a productive practice might have the following sequence:

1. First **warm up** by rhythmically swinging two or three clubs together. Get some readiness into your body by elevating the temperature of your muscles enough to make them responsive.

2. Start by hitting with a **middle iron**; a 5 or 6. Strike the first few balls with an easy — but not careless — swing. Right from the outset give attention to a correct grip, setup, and clubface alignment. Make your objective straight flight rather than any particular distance.

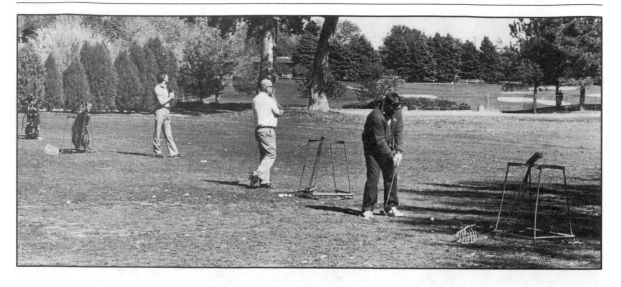

3. Then increase the **length** of your shots. Emphasize acceleration of the clubhead into the ball by concentrating on the rhythm of the swing.

4. Next, take a **longer iron,** hit a collection of balls, then hit a few with your longest iron or a high wood, and finally with your driver. Hit the driver for accuracy first, then let loose with your most powerful swings.

5. Now try some **placement hitting.** Select several different clubs, especially those you were least effective with last time on the course. Hit each one with a target awareness. Aim for a clump of grass, a leaf, a mound. Use each club to hit three different distances. Vary the trajectory. Work the ball, always being sensitive to the timing and rhythm of your swing. Experiment liberally, but keep asking yourself: What is the best club alignment? Ball position? Length of backswing? And so on.

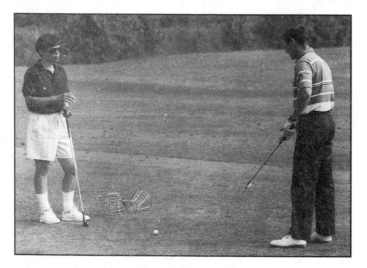

6. Try some **specialty shots.** A pitch and run with a 7-iron. Or a low punch shot with a 3-iron. Try for extra backspin with a wedge, or extra height with a 9-iron.

7. Then play a couple of **imaginary holes.** Use a course you are familiar with, and pretend you are playing specific holes. Hit the

drive, the approach shot, everything in succession as if you were actually on the course, and each shot in accordance with the position your previous shot would have put you in.

8. Finish the day with a club you feel **good** about, focusing particularly on the timing of your swing. That'll get you into the right frame of mind about the session and leave you with a positive reference for the next time on the course.

OTHER PRACTICE SITES

The range is not the only place where you can sharpen your golfing skills. Almost all courses will have a practice putting green. Many will also have

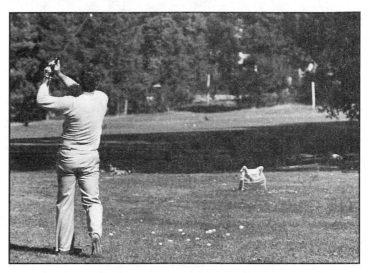

a practice sand trap. It's unlikely, however, to find a golf facility where you can rehearse shots from the rough or other difficult lies, but almost any vacant field will do for such practice. Parks or other open, grassy areas are potential places to hone your dexterity for pitching and chipping.

Additionally, obtain a supply of golf balls that have restricted flight. They will travel less distance, sometimes only half that of a regulation ball, so they can be hit with full swings in areas otherwise too confining. Or, when even less space is available, hit lightweight plastic balls from an old doormat. And don't forget the floor rug for putting practice. Besides, it's good therapy for breaking up a long study night.

Try par-3 courses. They're not only enjoyable and minimally time-consuming, they also focus attention on that most important part of golf, the short game.

Finally, there's no need to always use a ball for practice. You can make your pre-swing routine — grip, stance, and setup — more automatic on a rainy day at home. And you can set your timing and rhythm, along with a sense of balance, by simply swinging a club in the backyard. At the very least, swing a club for a few minutes every day. It maintains your sense of feel for the game and offers welcome relief from an otherwise technological existence.

● CREATING MUSCLE MEMORY

Practice makes perfect, it's often said. Not necessarily so. What practice does is make more **permanent** the things practiced. Accordingly, it's possible to practice **wrong** techniques, thereby making **flaws** more permanent. Every time you hit a ball, your body remembers, to some degree, the swing you took. So with each trial the characteristics of your swing become a bit more durably etched into your muscles until it's difficult to do it any other way. Consequently, it's vital to develop a "muscle memory" during practice, which is **technically correct, efficient,** and well programmed so it's **repeatable** on the course.

It's otherwise too easy, during practice, to slip into common habits such as a casual setup, poor weight distribution, or a lethargic clubhead. So try to hit each shot with the same measure of concentration as you do on the course, to the point where there's little difference between the two. Especially:

● Set up correctly, with proper alignment of grip, aim, stance, head position, and balance.

● Hit each shot with the ball at the optimal contact point in the arc of the swing.

● Be sure to get a full body turn in the windup, feeling extension in your arms.

● Initiate the downswing with the legs and hips.

● Hit forward and **through** the ball. Keep your clubhead active through the hitting zone, not letting it slow down until it comes to a natural rest after a complete flowing hit.

● Sense the rhythm of every swing.

Implant effective hitting patterns into your system so that out on the course your mind will be free of any mechanical thoughts about your swing. Develop the **feel** of your swing, and then when you need a crucial pitch shot to cross a stream and settle the ball onto a small green, all you need do is pull the appropriate neural memory switch and — click! Another perfect shot.

● FOR THE FUN OF IT

Although practice should be pursued with a reasonable degree of seriousness, it's also important to keep in perspective the primary purpose of golf: to enjoy playing. This is, after all, a **game.**

Make practice pleasurable. If it's drudgery, little benefit will emerge. There could even be some negative outcomes.

Add variety to the session. Use some time to experiment with small changes in your swing and note the effect. Hit deliberate fades, draws, other special shots. Even hit a few with no weight transfer, or with an inordinate flick of the wrists. In these whimsical moments your nervous system will still be reminded of what it takes to hit the ball well. You'll actually develop somewhat of a neural reference system that will sensitize your feedback to subtle differences in your swing that result in deviant ball flight. Thus you'll know the cause of an errant shot, and knowing the cause will automatically provide you with the cure.

The whole effect of adding diversion to the practice will be therapeutic, both mentally and physically. In the bargain you'll be reminded that golf is a sporting endeavor that, above all else, is to be enjoyed.

⬤ PRACTICE FOR THE BODY

Playing golf isn't the most physically excruciating thing you can do to yourself. But walking eighteen holes on a regulation course is nevertheless a fair bit of a hike — four miles or more. Carrying a set of clubs, or even dragging them along in a two-wheel pull-cart, adds to the strain. No wonder the nineteenth hole is so welcome.

To play your best golf you need to be responsive and unwavering — for the last holes as as well as the first. Thus your game could benefit and your scores potentially improve by attending to the following three areas of physical conditioning:

1.   Strength

Golf does not ask for raw, weightlifting-type brawn, but, rather, for occasions of explosive power. That calls for fluid, dynamic muscle contractions, not brute force.

Accordingly, resistance exercises will help prepare the body for hitting longer drives but only if the exercises concentrate on weight *training* instead of weight *lifting*. Weight training means using lighter weights and more repetitions than weight lifting. That'll produce the agile type of muscle readiness you can use to pull the trigger for the extra yards you may need to cross a stream traversing the fairway.

The upper body needs the most attention, particularly the shoulders and the back of the upper arms. Any workout with weights should:

⬤ be preceded by a warmup, including stretching,

● take the muscles through a full range of motion, and

● never be pushed to the point of strain.

2. Flexibility

When your muscles are supple and your joints flexible, you'll be more readily able to crank up your backswing for a full and unstrained body coil prior to hitting any shot. Even putting will be easier. So add some flexibility exercises to your regime, but keep in mind the basic rules about stretching:

● Do only static stretching. No bouncing! Curiously, bouncing works *against* the development of flexibility. So stretch *slowly*, and hold the end positions for a few seconds.

● Don't push to pain. If it hurts, stop. Increase your flexibility gradually, without forcing it, and the positions that are difficult to achieve now will be easy next week.

3. Endurance

When you climb up to an elevated tee on the eighteenth hole, your swing will still be intact and ready if your legs gave you no complaint about carrying you around the course. The best way to prepare your legs? Perhaps five-mile walks. But even better, take your body out for a jog three or four times a week. Join the countless others who jog just for the health of it. Your body will thank you.

Find jogging boring? Locate a circuit training course. That's a jogging trail with a series of marked stations, each one asking for a prescribed exercise at that station. The objective is to complete the circuit in as short a time as possible, or to increase the number of repetitions at each station whenever the course is run. It's a totally individualistic program because you set your own pace and determine your own number of repetitions. If you can't find an already established course, it's easy to create your own. Intersperse your jogging trip with frequent stops to do, for example, (1) trunk twisting, (2) bent-knee situps, (3) pushups, (4) squats to a half-sitting position, (5) alternately raising knees to your chest, (6) heel raises while standing with toes on the edge of a step, (7) raising legs while lying flat on your back, (8) pushups off ground and clap hands in between each pushup, and (9) jumping and reaching as high as you can.

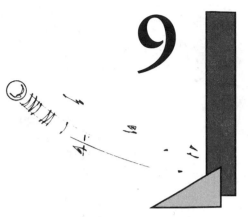

Strategy for the Course

"Ah, the game's the thing!" according to an old Shakespearean philosophy-of-the-pub. It means that all the talk and thought and practice are unfulfilled until a player's acquired skills can be tested on the real stage of competition. Going through the motions without the emotions is only a halfway house. Golf is, after all, designed to be **played**.

And there's **strategy** to the playing. It might not seem there is, or needs to be, since the purpose of the game — to get the ball from here to there in the least number of attempts — is very direct. But the encumbrance is that no two golf courses, no two fairways, no two lies, are exactly alike. There are nuances of terrain and trees and grass and sand and wind and weather. So on its journey to its final resting place, the ball can put a golfer through trials of patience and fiendish frustrations and vast resolutions and illusions of grandeur that ebb and sway with each new shot. It's why golf can compel one into a complete commitment of the psyche.

Happily, two things are in the golfer's favor. First, the competition is essentially with the course, not an opponent, so the design of play is resolved by the lie of each ball. Second, the pace of the game is such that there's no pressure to make split-second decisions. There's time to reason, to calculate, to intelligently reckon every situation. Thus the game appeals also to a mathematical mind, for shot selection is based on laws of probability for success. In all, it asks the golfer to be a resourceful strategist.

THE FIRST LAW: PLAY POSITION GOLF

Start with the most basic of all strategies: **keep the ball in play**. Hitting a long ball is impressive, but not when it occurs at the expense of accuracy.

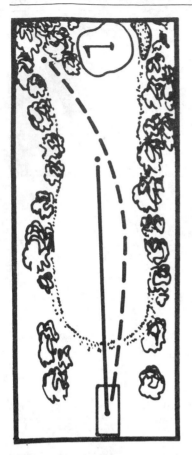

It's better to hit a controlled ball that finishes in position to make the next shot easier. A long drive that finishes in the rough compounds the difficulty of the next shot. A shorter drive that leaves a clean fairway lie is more accommodating. So play **position** golf. Make accuracy your objective, for all eighteen holes and for every shot. Think ahead to give yourself the advantage of landing each ball so that the next shot can be struck without the interference of a hazard.

NEVER HURRY THE OPENING SHOT

On the first tee you'll probably be anxious, your muscles still tight. There are other groups, waiting their turn, watching you tee up. The first drive is eventful. Smack it well and you're suddenly relaxed, optimistic. Hit it poorly and it's an aggravating start. It's important not to rush this opening shot. Don't hurry your preparation just to get it over with. Be completely ready. Take some easy practice swings, a few deep breaths. Gain control of your heightened state. Be deliberate. Set up correctly, double check it. Fix your eyes intently on the ball, emphasize the smoothness and completeness of your backswing, and strike the ball for accurate flight rather than distance.

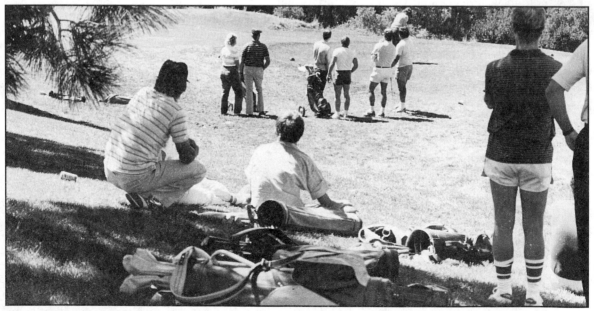

TEE THE BALL PROPERLY

How high to tee the ball for a drive? Generally, with its equator about the same height as the top of a driver sitting flat on the ground. Be wary of the common suggestion to tee the ball low when hitting into a wind and high when hitting with a trailing wind. Your main thought, always, is to peg the ball at a height that allows for solid impact. On short holes, don't copy other players' propensity for hitting the ball from the ground. Teeing the ball provides a margin of error so you're less likely to catch too much turf. Sit the ball a quarter inch above the ground for a short iron; a half inch for a long iron.

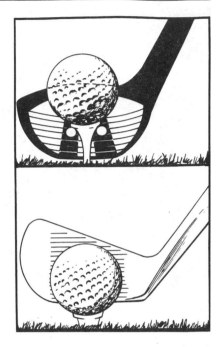

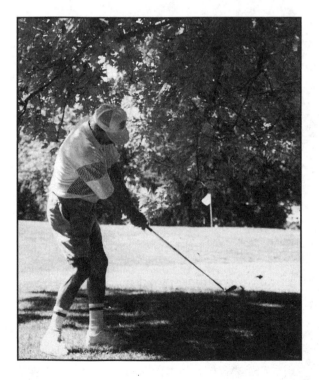

PLAY THE SAFEST SHOT

Always look for the safest route to the green. This isn't always the shortest route. This is often true when you're in the predicament of having an obstacle, such as trees, between your ball and the green. Should you try to rifle the ball through the trees and risk it catching the woodwork? It depends on how you feel at the moment. But it also depends on logic. Is there enough of an opening? And is there another potential hazard lurking even if you do get through? The best choice is to swallow your sense of gambling and find a safe way out of the trees so your next shot can be hit from a clear fairway lie.

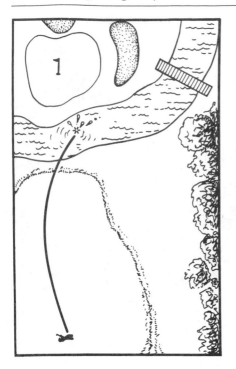

STAY AWAY FROM TROUBLE

Whenever there is potential trouble ahead, hit away from it. For instance, if there are trees along one side of the fairway but not the other, target your shot for the open side where there's more room for error. The same decision applies when aiming for a green that's guarded by sand traps on one side only. Or, if there's a water hazard crossing the fairway ahead and you think your best of shots could clear it, consider laying the ball up short instead of risking a penalty stroke for plopping in the drink. Be realistic about your chances, and about your ability. Always ask if the possible results are worth the risk. Give every shot a margin for error.

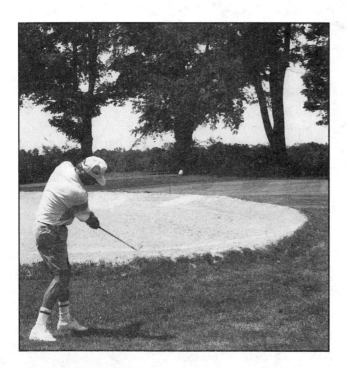

PLAN AHEAD

Strategy can never be myopic. Any plan must appraise not only what manner of shot is needed for the immediate situation but also whether the result will leave the ball playable for the **next** shot. For example, say you have yourself locked into a tight lie next to an imposing sand trap, and the pin is tucked in just beyond the trap. If you try to chip for the pin but instead dump the ball into the trap, you will have magnified the predicament. The objective should be to park the ball somewhere on the green, even if that means hitting away from the hole. But the reward is that your next stroke will be a putt, not a sand shot.

POSITION THE BALL WISELY

Most courses have at least one hole with a dog-leg; a bend in the fairway. These diabolical detours often have the bend at less than a driver's length away, and the corner is usually heavy with trees. The first impulse might be to go over the trees to short-cut the corner. But that's too risky. The next thought could be to lay the ball just around the corner. But even if you have that kind of pinpoint accuracy, a surprise often awaits when you find that the next shot must still bypass some of the woods. Answer: Stay clear of the corner. Get the ball out in the open where there's plenty of working room for the next shot.

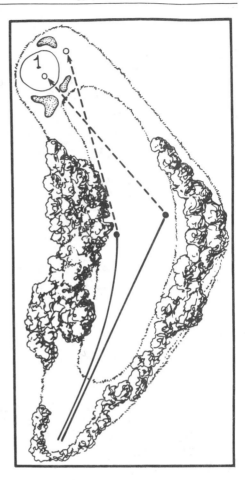

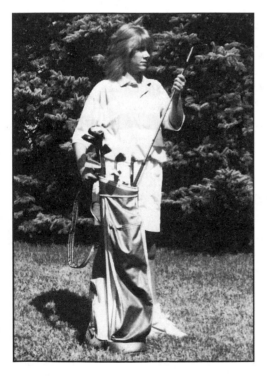

USE ENOUGH CLUB

When you get to know from experience how far you normally hit with each club, use that information as a constant reference, especially as you approach the green. Look for objects that can help you judge the needed distance, such as trees or other players near the green, and the flagstick itself. Having made your appraisal, be sure to choose enough club. Beware of the tendency to "underclub" by selecting a weapon that requires you to hit full-out to reach the target. Choose instead a club that will get you there with a smooth swing of less than maximum effort. Always use rhythm over muscle for your approach shots.

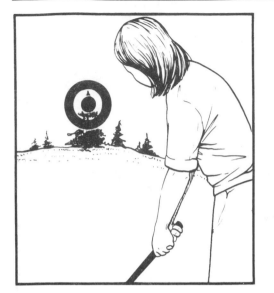

HAVE A SPECIFIC TARGET

Never hit a careless shot. Always have a specific target. Identify a place where you want the ball to go. Do it for **every shot**. Sometimes it's neglected. Say you're on a dog-leg and all you want to do is lay the ball somewhere in the bend. Or suppose you're on a tee with a vast ranchland of open fairway in front of you. It's too easy to hit a random shot, without specific direction. Instead, pick out **something** as a reference for aiming. Then mentally focus on that aim point. This will get you into a more careful alignment and give your swing directional purpose. It will also zero your attention on the target rather than on any potential hazards lurking nearby.

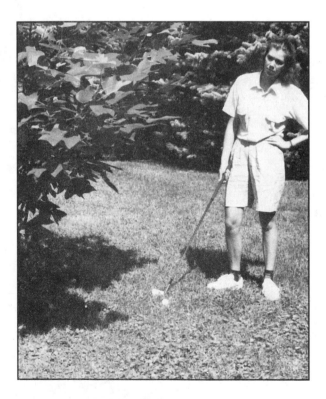

PLAY WITHIN YOUR ABILITY

It is sometimes tempting to try to pull off a dazzling "miracle" shot that will extricate you from a precarious situation or otherwise would give you a psychological uplift. The lure arises when you need to get out of a perilous hazard, or when you need an infinitely accurate shot to go through some trees, or when you simply want to out-hit everyone from the tee. But always ask yourself: What would you **like** to happen, and what are you capable of **making** happen? Base your decision on an honest judgment of your ability. Keep in mind that you are playing essentially against the **course**, not other players.

STAY WITH YOUR NATURAL FLIGHT

No sense in arguing with your natural flight character. For instance, if you normally slice the ball moderately to the right, don't align yourself to hit straight down the fairway hoping that this time you'll drill the ball true. Aim off to the left and allow the ball to take its natural curving flight back to the target. Or, as another example, if you never get much backspin on your chip shots, aim short of the target and allow for the roll instead of hoping that this time your chip shot will "sit down" next to the pin. The basis of accuracy is repetition, not experimentation, particularly as it averages out over a round of play.

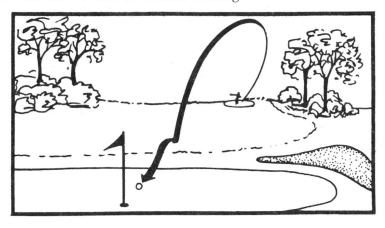

ATTEND TO THE SWING, NOT THE LIE

Here's your chance to be cool. Say your ball has rolled up next to an obstacle and your swing for the next shot will be restricted. Neurotic players become so mentally affixed to the obstacle that they forget the ball. They swing primarily to avoid the obstacle rather than to hit the ball. Keep your concentration — take time to consider the situation, and try enough practice swings to measure your clearance. When you know how far you can take the club back, put the information in your neural system, then ignore the obstacle and attend to the swing you just rehearsed. See the positive result, then congratulate yourself for staying mentally collected.

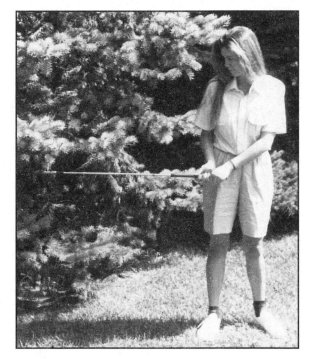

⌐• NEVER THREE PUTT

Make this vow: you'll never three-putt a green. Help keep your promise by habitually reading the greens early, while you're still approaching from

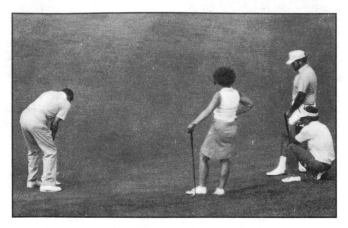

the fairway. Watch the roll of your approach shot if it finishes on the putting green to get some information about the lay of the surface. Get an additional reading by watching the putts of other players. Survey the terrain from several different vantage points. Then maintain this basic philosophy: Never leave a short putt short of the hole; but on long putts expand the target to a circle around the hole, and hit the first putt to finish inside that circle, then sink the next putt.

⌐• MAKE ONLY INTELLIGENT MISTAKES

In summary, an overall strategy is to limit your mistakes to those you make with your body, not with your brain. Always choose a logical route

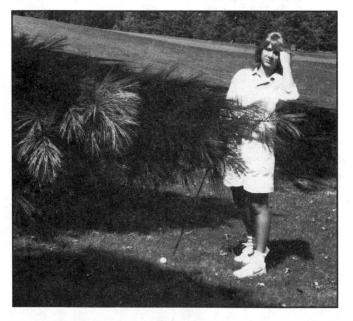

to the green. Hit only shots that have a high probability for success. You especially need mental calm and a sense of reason if you hit an errant shot that leaves you with an awful lie. There will be emotional overrun, and out of frustration you may try for a miraculous recovery shot. But you've probably never practiced the shot you'd need, and the results might only redouble the unfortunate situation. So stay logical. Keep the percentages in your favor. Play only intelligent golf.

10

The Mental Game

Mind and body are not separate. Mental and physical phenomena are interrelated, each dependent on the other and each influencing the other. That's well known. It becomes explicitly apparent, sometimes painfully so, on the golf course. The game can seize a person's emotions so completely as to make it sometimes difficult to distinguish whether the ball was hit with one's body or one's brain. It's because performance on the course is often a product of one's state of mind. How you feel on the inside will be reflected by how you do on the outside. If you feel alive, energetic, and confident, your shots will have vivid resolution. But if you're nervous, frustrated, and angry, your play will be erratic. Here are some ways to help you mobilize the proper mental states conducive to optimal play.

BEFORE THE START OF PLAY

It's common to feel a generalized state of anxiety before you tee up the first ball. How well will you play today? Might you be embarrassed in front of your friends? Will you be paired up with strangers? Will there be a lot of other golfers watching you hit your opening drive?

Whatever the source, some pre-round apprehension is universal. To some degree, **everyone** feels it: the pros, the club player, the occasional weekender. To help dissipate this trepidation, before you walk up to the first tee, try the following:

Think Constructively

Rid your mind of negative thoughts. Think instead of the skills you know you have. Visually picture them. See yourself doing well. There's only a given amount of room in your brain. Fill the space with constructive thoughts, and they'll crowd out the negative ones.

Be Honest with Yourself

Admit that there is, after all, only so much you're capable of doing. Make up your mind that you're going to play within the capabilities you have, not trying anything you haven't yet acquired in your hitting repertoire.

Create Positive Energy

Collect positive vibrations. Feel alive. Be optimistic. Sense the very enjoyment of being able to play. Forge an upbeat emotional tone that will stimulate your game. Put on your own headset and talk your brain into a positive state of reference.

Be Physically Ready

Go to the practice putting green. Hit a variety of putts, including the short ones you always expect to make on the course. If there is an allowable place, hit some short chip shots. And if there is a practice range, consider hitting a small basket of balls. At the very least, loosen up your muscles with stretching and rhythmical swinging to set your timing.

Treat it as a Game

This is a game, the purpose of which is to reduce stress, not create it. Golf should add enjoyment to your day, not frustration. Get caught up with the pure, unadulterated pleasure of playing. With the proper mental attitude, golf will be a stimulant to your psyche, not a depressant.

PLAY POSITIVE GOLF

Arnold Palmer, golfer extraordinaire, once said that when he hit a perfect shot, he was never surprised, because that's exactly what he **wanted** to do. He was only surprised, he said, when the ball did **not** go where he was aiming.

By contrast, it's common to find weekend players expressing amazement at the unexpected good fortune of having their ball go where they wanted it to. Some golfers have a sense of impending doom, and when they hit a poor shot, they treat it as a reconfirmation of their inadequate ability. They prepare for a shot by thinking, usually subconsciously, that they will not strike the ball well. As a result, their swing lacks determination.

Watch golf champions. There is confidence in their every manner — the way they step up to the ball, the conviction in their swing, even their irk when the ball does not fly exactly true. They have an encompassing belief in their ability to play excellent golf, especially under pressure. They are intensely self-assured. It's the only way they **can** feel. They could not perform at top level if they did not have supreme confidence in their skills.

While you are (probably) not entertaining the thought of becoming a pro golfer, you nevertheless do want to play as well as you can. At the very least, you want to have enough capability to keep from chasing ball after ball into a hazard.

So act confident, even if it's an **act**. Your body will respond to your mental attitudes. Tell it positive things. Believe that you are capable. Think success. Play psychological games with yourself to stay poised, assured, and decisive. Then crush your drives with a free swing. Swat your approach shots with conviction. And spank your putts confidently. When the ball goes where you wanted it to, you'll never be surprised.

▮• FOCUS ON THE TARGET, NOT A HAZARD

Sound strategy is to always hit away from trouble. When there is a lurking hazard, pick out a safe target — one that provides a margin for error if you stray from your point of aim. Then focus intently on that **target**, and blank out the hazard. Overconsciousness of a hazard can create muscle tension and force you into trying to "steer" the ball away from the obstacle rather than hitting it normally.

Here's a common scenario. A golfer is confronted with a water hazard that could be crossed with a good tee shot. Lacking confidence, the golfer pulls out an old ball, tees it up higher than usual, and swings in the manner of trying to knock an apple out of a tree. Predictable result? The ball probably gets dunked into the water anyhow. The hazard has become a magnet.

Once you have identified where you want to send the ball, mentally rehearse the shot. Don't start your swing until you have **seen** the result. Then put on your mental blinders. Instead of being mesmerized by the hazard and letting it influence your swing, think only of the target. Say to the ball, "Go there!"

▙● PROFIT FROM YOUR MISTAKES

Every golfer makes mistakes. It's what you do **after** a mistake that is important. When you hit a poor shot, you could react in one of two ways. You could respond negatively by getting angry, frustrated, or discrediting yourself. Or you could immediately seek a positive solution to **why** you made the mistake. For example, if you realize you sliced the ball because you kept your weight on your back foot, then remind yourself to have a proper transfer of weight for upcoming shots. This way you'll be attending to the **remedy** for your flaw instead of brooding over the flaw itself. Your mistake can actually be used to reinforce something positive about your swing. So think of what you could have done better, and perhaps take a few rehearsal swings when you realize the origin of the faulty shot so you can desensitize your nerves to the flaw and re-program the correct motion. It'll help for the next shot, and also help you to enjoy the game more.

▙● PLAY EACH SHOT AS AN ENTITY

Mistakes seem to happen in clusters. One bad shot is followed by another, and another.

The worst mistake is to follow a mistake with another mistake. If a shot disobeyed your orders, don't let that forecast another bad shot. If you fume over the error, it could transfer into the next shot. Golf is a difficult game to play when you're emotional. Your brain may still know what to do, but your obstinate body won't respond if your provoked psyche gets in the way.

Use **selective attention**. Focus attention only on what is relevant for your performance. What **is** relevant is the rhythm and timing of your swing. What **isn't** relevant is the previous shot. Isolate on each swing. When you hit a poor shot, remind yourself of what to do to make the next one better, and then self-talk confidence back into your attitude. Walk away from the previous shot, both physically and mentally. As you approach the ball for your next shot, build up your positive concentration. Plan the shot. Be sure to take some practice swings. Don't hit the ball until you're ready, not only with your swing but also with your mind. Sense the rhythm of the stroke you're about to hit. Selectively attend to the present.

Try this technique: Play each shot as if it were the only one you'll hit that day. That way you'll focus on one shot at a time, and collectively it will add up to a higher level of concentration for the whole round.

▌● PLAY THE COURSE, NOT YOUR OPPONENT

Maybe you have a friendly agreement with the others in your playing group that the highest score for the day will buy the beverages at the end of the round. Or you and another player might be partners competing against two other players. But it's always the **course** that is your biggest challenge. So concentrate on your own game, not anyone else's. It's especially critical when other players can consistently outdistance you from the tee. That's a psychological edge, and it may compel you into trying to force some extra yardage out of your driver. But if you keep your sense of logic and play position golf, that will be your most economical decision in the long run. At the end of the day, whether you had the lowest score or not, you'll know you played your best against the natural challenge of the course.

▌● HOW TO MENTALLY PRACTICE THIS GAME

There is a widely used mental tool in sports that incorporates the mind's lucid capacity for imagination. Through a technique of visual dramatization called **mental practice,** an athlete will, while in a state of quietude, create a mental image of his/her own performance, trying in the process to generate all the sensations and environmental conditions of the skill, including the actual feel of the performance. It is a virtual dreamland of rehearsal.

Research has shown rather conclusively that using mental practice in combination with overt physical practice can produce greater improvements in performance than either method used alone. Here are some general guidelines for using mental practice:

1. Choose a time and place where you can be undisturbed.

2. Close your eyes, breathe deeply, and relax as completely as possible. Feel your muscles go limp.

3. Clear your mind. Imagine a blank white screen. Think of emptiness. Free your mind of all thoughts.

4. Visualize yourself hitting the ball, including all aspects of the event. For example, if you are rehearsing a drive, see yourself stepping up to the ball, addressing it, setting your sights, and so on, right through the flight and landing of the shot.

5. Visualize in color, making the colors as vivid as you can.

6. Try to **feel** the movement of the swing. Create the very physical sensations of the performance.

7. Use all your senses. Not only should you see and feel the skills of the game, but you should also hear the sound of impact with the ball or distracting noises such as passing traffic. Imagine the heat of a mid-summer day, or the crisp air of an autumn morning. Even try to smell the scent of new-mown grass.

8. Include the presence of other players in your visual game.

9. Mentally practice all elements of the game, including short chip shots and putting.

10. Rehearse the proper emotional climate of the game, in particular seeing yourself in full command of your psyche to prepare for and hit a recovery shot following an errant ball.

11. Sometimes visualize in slow motion, trying to be critically analytical of your skill during these slowed-down performances.

12. Keep the sessions reasonably short. Several brief rehearsal periods are better than one prolonged session.

Mental practice is a valuable complement to your skill. It can be used not only to improve your ability but also to program your swing when you're on the course. Before hitting a shot, you can visualize the whole event, in the process generating the proper muscular readiness for the swing. Thus you can actually **see** each shot before you hit it, and then merely let your body act out the swing you mentally rehearsed. Use visualization often, both during quiet times and out on the course. Go see the movie that's in your head.

Golf Exercises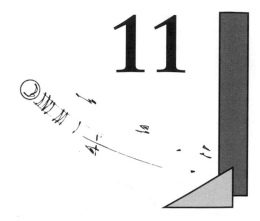

Hitting a golf ball is not the most physically demanding thing you'll ever do, but hitting a golf ball **well** requires supple muscles and a responsive body. A properly prepared nerve-muscle machinery will enable you to swing the club more freely and hit more convincingly. Therefore, each practice session will be more profitable and each time on the course more invigorating.

Moreover, golf is a sport of composure. It cannot be successfully played when your muscles are tight. To acquire the skills of the game, and ultimately to play with flair, requires a mind-body attitude of permissiveness. Your inner self must be free to hit with expressive quality, always in the proper state of control to execute a swing of appropriate rhythm and power. So your muscles must be calm to start, yet ready for a vigorous thrust of energy. At other times they must remain calm for the deft touch of a short spank of the ball.

Thus, the game requires of your body some strength, some endurance, and good flexibility. To play your best golf, you need to be alive and unwavering — for the last holes as well as the first.

It starts with ready strength. Golf does not ask for raw, weight-lifting-type of brawn, but rather for occasions of explosive power. That calls for fluid, dynamic muscle contractions, not brute force.

Then there is the hike. Walking eighteen holes on a regulation course is four miles or more and the weight of the clubs imposes additional strain.

For an unhindered swing, you need flexibility. When your muscles are elastic and your joints are limber, you'll be more readily able to crank up your swing for a full and unconstrained strike of the ball. Even putting will be easier.

⬤ FLEXIBILITY

On any day, before you hit a golf ball, do the following stretching exercises. They will limber your muscles and joints and reduce the potential for a muscle pull or strain. Do each one several times. Stretch **slowly**, and hold the end position for a few seconds.

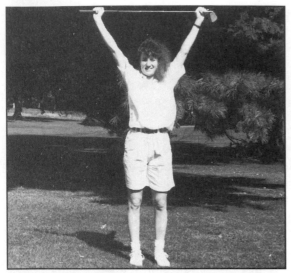

Hold the club in front of you, belt high, then raise to this position. Keep your arms straight throughout.

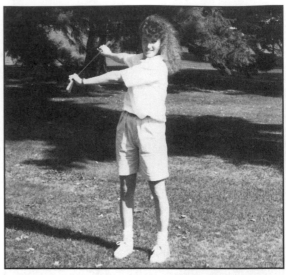

With the club again held in front of you, twist to each side, giving your spine as much turn as possible.

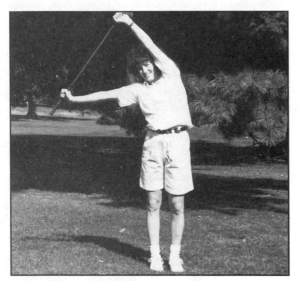

Now take the club overhead, bend to each side, and hold your head steady as you go.

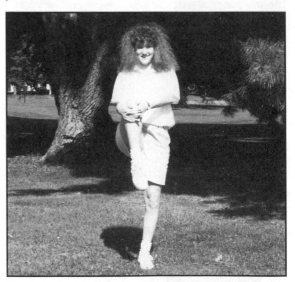

Finish with this modified knee-lift, alternating sides and pulling your knee well into your chest.

▌. STRENGTH

With power in readiness, you'll be able to pull the trigger for the extra yards you may need to drive over a stream traversing the fairway, or at least be in front of everyone else. By using the club to help you develop power, you can also educate your body to the task.

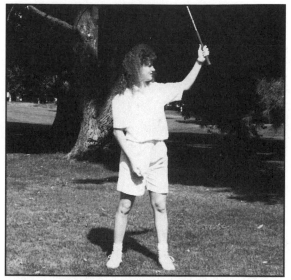

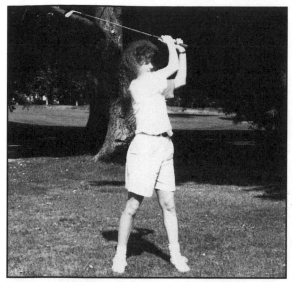

After warming up, swing the club vigorously, non-stop. Add weight to the clubhead if you can.

Now use single-handed swings, one hand then the other, to strengthen each side of the body.

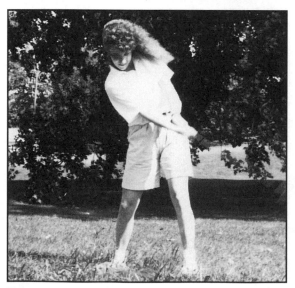

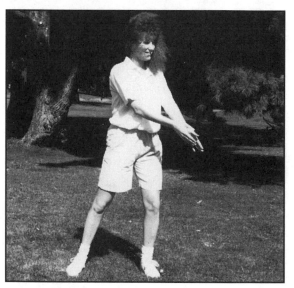

Take an old club, find a pasture, and cut some grass by drilling the club through the high vegetation.

Pull your left arm toward a swing while you resist with your right. Then push right against left.

● ENDURANCE

When you climb up to an elevated tee on the eighteenth hole, your swing will still be intact and ready if your legs gave you no complaint about carrying you around the course. Your club will still have the electricity it needs at the end if you have prepared your endurance.

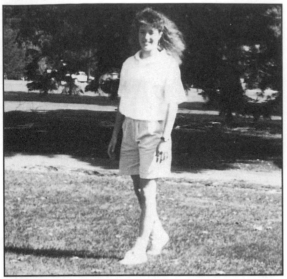

Golf is a walking sport. Prepare by taking a five-mile walk three or four times a week.

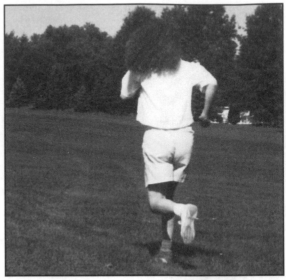

Better yet, take yourself out for a jog. Your golf will be livelier and your body will thank you.

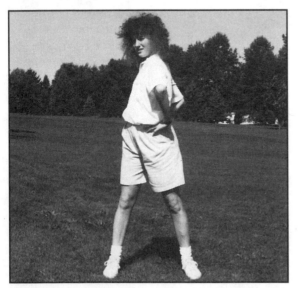

Add variety to jogging by interspersing it with trunk twisting, push-ups, half-squats, sit-ups, etc.

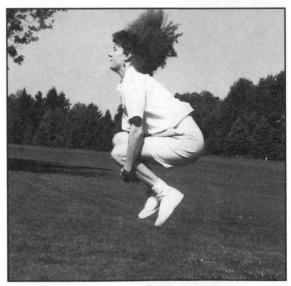

Add spring to your legs with "rabbit-jumps," repeated rapidly in succession until tired.

Glossary of Golf Terms

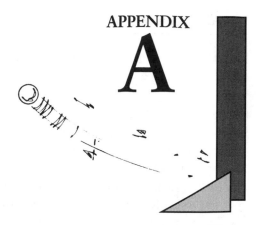

Become a golf linguist, so you can effectively communicate on the links, at the 19th hole, or during a lawn party following a tournament. It is also helpful for understanding the rules, which are presented in the next section of this appendix.

Ace A hole completed in one stroke. A hole-in-one.

Address Position assumed by a player at the ball before beginning the swing.

Approach Shot A medium or short iron shot (except when hit from the teeing area) which is intended to have the ball finish on the putting green.

Apron The perimeter grass around the putting green which is not cut as short as the green, but shorter than the fairway grass. Also called the "fringe," or "collar;" less commonly, "frog hair."

Away The ball which, at any time after all players have hit their shots in turn, is farthest away from the hole, and thus is next in turn to play.

Back Door A putted ball which rolls around the perimeter of the hole and then, when it appears it will stay out, drops in the back of the hole.

Back Nine The second nine holes of an 18-hole golf course.

Backspin The backward spin imparted to a ball to make it "bite," or stop quickly.

Ball Marker A small coin or other small disc used to spot the position of a ball on the green.

Banana Ball Slang for a shot that curves emphatically from left to right. A slice.

Best-Ball A match in which one golfer competes against the better ball (the best score) of two other players on each hole; or, the best ball of three other players. (The term is commonly misapplied to "four-ball" matches.)

Birdie A score of one stroke under par for a hole.

Bite Action of a ball having sufficient backspin to make it stop quickly, or actually bounce and roll backwards, upon landing (usually refers to a landing on the putting green).

Blind Hole One on which the flagstick cannot be seen by a golfer hitting a drive or an approach shot.

Bogey A score of one stroke over par for a hole.

Brassie An old, original term for the No. 2 wood.

Break   The slant or slope of a putting green; also, the sideward curve of a putt as it rolls on the green.

Bunker   A prepared area of ground, usually a hollow, from which turf has been removed and replaced with sand. The term is used synonymously with "sand trap."

Caddie   Someone who carries a player's clubs and may assist that player as the rules provide.

Carry   The distance a ball travels in the air before landing.

Casual Water   Any temporary accumulation of water on the course which is not a normal water hazard. Dew is not casual water.

Chip Shot   A short approach shot to the green.

Closed Face   Clubface which is aimed left of the intended line of flight either at address or on impact.

Closed Stance   Address position where the left foot is closer than the right foot to the intended line of flight.

Clubface   Normal striking surface of the clubhead.

Collar   Perimeter grass around a green or the edges of a hazard.

Course   The whole area within which play is permitted.

Cup   Metal or plastic lining fitted into the hole.

Divot   A piece of turf lifted out by a player's clubhead during a swing.

Dog-Leg   A bend in the fairway either to the right or left.

Dormie   When a player, or side in match play, is ahead as many holes as remain to be played in the match.

Double Bogey   A score of two strokes over par for a hole.

Double Eagle   A score of three strokes under par for a hole.

Down   The number of strokes or holes a player or team is behind an opponent.

Draw   A shot that starts on the intended line of flight and then curves slightly to the left.

Drive   A shot hit with a driver from the teeing area.

Driver   The No. 1 wood.

Drop   The act of putting a ball into play in accordance with the rules whereby a player stands erect, holds the ball at shoulder height and arm's length, and drops it, thereupon to be played as it lies.

Duck Hook   A shot that curves sharply to the left and abruptly nosedives to the ground.

Duffer   Slang term for a poor golfer.

Eagle   A score of two strokes under par for a hole.

Explosion Shot   Hitting out of a sand trap and displacing a spray of sand with the club.

Fade   A shot that starts on the intended line of flight and then curves slightly to the right.

Fairway   The specially prepared, closely cropped area of ground intended for play between the tee and the putting green.

Fat Shot   Unintentionally striking the ground behind the ball during a swing.

Flagstick   A removable straight indicator, with or without bunting or other material attached, centered in the hole to show its position.

Fore   A call used to warn those in danger of being hit by a ball.

Forward Press   Subtle movement, usually of the hands, more or less toward the target immediately prior to starting the back swing.

Four-Ball   A match in which two golfers play as a team against two other golfers, and each team counts only the better ball of the two players as their score for each hole. Often incorrectly called "best-ball."

Foursome   A group of four players.

Fringe   *See* "apron."

Front Nine   The first nine holes of an 18-hole golf course.

Gimme   Slang term for a putt so short it is conceded to an opponent.

Green   The putting surface; that area of closely cut grass containing the hole, cup, and flagstick.

Green Fee   The money paid for the privilege of playing a course.

Grounding The Club   Placing the sole of the club on the ground in preparation for starting a backswing.

Halved or Halving a Hole   In match play, to tie a hole, each side achieving the same score.

Handicap   The number of artificial strokes a player receives to adjust his or her scoring ability, usually based on that golfer's best scores from a given number of recent rounds, and used to equate players of differential ability for a tournament.

Hazard   In general it means any natural obstacle on the course, although the rules recognize only bunkers and water (except casual water) as hazards.

Hole   The objective; a round receptacle in the green, four inches in diameter.

Hole-High   A shot to a green that finishes even with the hole but off to one side.

Hole-In-One   Completing a hole in only one stroke. An "ace."

Hole Out   To make a stroke that puts the ball into the cup.

Honor   The right to drive or play first from a teeing area, determined by the lower score on the preceding hole, or on the first tee by choice of the players.

Hook   A shot that curves from right to left during its flight.

Iron   Any club with a head made primarily of metal, but not including putters or woods with metal heads.

LPGA   Ladies Professional Golf Association.

Lag   A putt played primarily to finish near the hole rather than actually in it.

Lie   The finishing position of a ball after a shot. Also, the number of strokes taken at that point for a hole. (For example, a golfer having taken three strokes is said to "lie 3.")

Links   Another term for a golf course. Originally it meant a seaside.

Lip   The rim of the hole, or of a bunker.

Loft   The degree to which a clubface lies back from vertical.

Mashie   An old, original term for a 5-iron.

Match Play   Competition in which each hole is a separate contest, the lowest score winning that hole, and the winner of the match being the player or side winning the most holes.

Medal Play   Antiquated term for competition based on the total number of strokes taken for the match. Correct term is "stroke play."

Mulligan   A second attempt at a shot that was not to a player's liking, permitted in a social game by mutual agreement of the players, and usually granted on the first tee. Not recognized by the rules of golf.

Nassau   A scoring system of granting one point for the lowest total strokes for the front nine, another point for the lowest score on the back nine, and a third point for the lowest total score for the entire 18.

Niblick   An old, original term for a 9-iron.

Nineteenth Hole   Euphemistic term for the golf course's barroom.

Open Face   Clubface which is aimed right of the intended line of flight either at address or on impact.

Open Stance   Address position where the right foot is closer than the left foot to the intended line of flight.

Open Tournament   Competition in which both amateurs and professionals are eligible.

Out of Bounds   Ground on which play is prohibited.

Overclubbing   Hitting with a lower number club than needed. Example: using an 8-iron when a 9-iron would have provided the distance needed.

PGA   Professional Golfer's Association.

Par   The number of strokes a good player should need to play a hole without mistake under ordinary conditions, always allowing two putts on the green.

Penalty Stroke   A stroke added to the score of a player for certain infractions of the rules.

Pin-High   *See* "hole high."

Pitch Shot   A medium-length shot of high trajectory to the green.

Pitch-And-Run   A shot played with low trajectory, intended to gain most of its distance by roll rather than by flight. Occasionally called "bump and run."

Pitching Wedge   An iron that is second only to the sand wedge in its degree of loft.

Play Through   An invitation by a slower-playing group to allow the following group to hit and "play through" as the slow group waits.

Preferred Lies   *See* "winter rules."

Provisional Ball   A second ball played from the same spot as the original when the first ball is suspected to be lost or out of bounds.

Pull   A shot that travels on a more or less straight path but to the left of the intended line of flight.

Push   A shot that travels on a more or less straight path but to the right of the intended line of flight.

Putt   Stroke made on the green with a putter.

Putting Green   Technically, the ground of the hole which is specially prepared for putting, but liberally referring to the putting area itself.

Reading the Green   Determining the line that a shot (usually a putt) will probably take on the green.

Rough   The area bordering the fairway where the grass, weeds, etc., are allowed to grow freely.

Round   The playing of the holes of a course, usually meaning eighteen total.

Rub of the Green   An unpredictable happening when a ball in motion or at rest is stopped or deflected by a source which is not a normal part of the course or a hazard thereof.

Ryder Cup   Competition between men's professional teams from Great Britain and Europe against the United States team.

Sand Trap   Common term for a bunker. A hazard filled with sand.

Sand Wedge   The iron with the greatest loft, specially designed for play from a sand trap.

Scratch Player   A player who has a handicap of zero, earned through consistent play near par.

Scuff   To hit the ground before the ball on the downswing.

Setup   *See* "address."

Shank   To contact the ball with the neck of the club instead of the face.

Short Game   Combined strokes of pitching, chipping, and putting.

Slice   A shot that curves from left to right during flight.

Spoon   Old, original term for the No. 3 wood.

Stance   Position of the feet when addressing the ball.

Stroke Play   Competition in which the total strokes taken for the round (or rounds) are used to determine the winner.

Summer Rules   Term sometimes used to describe play which disallows "winter rules." In effect it means to play the ball as it lies.

Target Line   An imaginary line from the ball direct to the intended target or objective.

Tee   The peg by which the ball is elevated before striking it from the teeing ground or, the teeing ground itself.

Tee Markers   Two markers placed on the teeing ground to indicate the forward limits allowed for setting the ball in preparation for hitting.

Tee Shot   The first shot played on a hole.

Teeing Ground   The designated starting place for the hole to be played.

Texas Wedge   An expression referring to the use of a putter to play a ball not on the green.

Top   To hit the ball above its center with the bottom of the clubface.

Underclubbing   Using a club that will not provide enough distance for the desired shot.

USGA   United States Golf Association.

Up   The number of strokes or holes a player or team is ahead of an opponent.

Up and Down   Holing out in two strokes from off the green, but often loosely applied to approach shots and putting.

Waggle   Preliminary movement of the clubhead and/or the golfer prior to starting the swing.

Winter Rules   A local rule granted by a course which is not in top playable condition and the players are therefore allowed to improve the lie of their ball.

Wood   A club with the head made primarily of wood, or, having the configuration and clubhead mass of a wood.

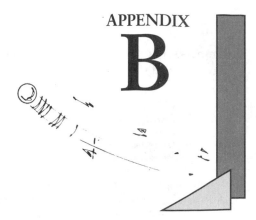

The Rules Simplified

The first written rules of golf were set down in 1744 to govern play on that most venerable of all courses, St. Andrews, in Scotland. There were only thirteen of those early regulations and they included, curiously, an allowance for players to subtract strokes from their own score when an opponent violated certain of the rules.

Today the rules of golf are administered jointly by two organizations: The United States Golf Association and The Royal and Ancient Golf Club of St. Andrews, Scotland. In their full treatise they read with the literary ease of a life insurance policy. What follows here is a condensed version of the situations most likely to occur on the course.

THE FIRST RULE: COURTESY ON THE COURSE

Certain unwritten rules have, over the years, become established as the expected sporting behavior for all participants in golf. Especially the following:

- So that each player might have full concentration for their shot, no one should talk, move, or stand close to or directly behind the ball or the hole when a player is addressing the ball or making a stroke.

- In the interest of all, players should play without delay. If a group of players fails to keep pace on the course and falls behind to where there is at least one clear hole in front of them, that group should allow the group behind them to pass and "play through."

- Players searching for a lost ball should signal the group behind them to play through as soon as it becomes apparent the ball will not be found easily.

- When a player's ball is on the wrong fairway, the players on that fairway have the right of way and should be permitted to hit without interruption or delay.

- All players must have their own set of clubs to play a course.

- Before leaving a bunker, a player should fill in and smooth over all footprints and other depressions.

- A player should replace and press down any turf cut by the swing of a club (i.e., divot), or repair any marks made on the green by a ball, spiked shoes, or anything else.

- Use the call of "fore" as a warning to other players who are in danger of being struck by a ball.

● On par-3 holes, it is common for golfers who have reached the putting green to invite players of the following group to hit their tee shots, during which time the waiting group should stand to one side of the green.

● No golf bags or clubs other than the putter should be carried onto the green.

● When all players are on the green, the player who is closest to the hole should attend the flagstick, removing it upon request of the player about to putt or when the putted ball is on its way.

● When attending the flagstick, stand to one side of the hole, at arm's length, and hold the stick in readiness for its removal.

● When marking the position of a ball on the green, place a small coin or marker behind the ball. If the marker will be in another player's line of putt, place the marker the necessary putterhead lengths to one side.

● No player should stand so that their shadow falls over another player's line of putt.

● When the play of a hole is completed, players should immediately leave the putting green. Scores for the hole should be recorded after leaving the green.

● And of course, clubs are instruments designed for hitting the ball, not for tossing in anger.

METHODS OF SCORING

Basically, there are two ways to score in golf, and thereby to create competition: match play and stroke play. In match play, each hole becomes a separate contest, the winner of the hole being the player (or side, if players are paired into teams) that finishes that hole in the fewest strokes. The winner of the match is the player (or side) winning the most holes for the round. In this method of scoring a hole can be **halved** if each side (or the competing players) takes the same number of strokes, and thus there is no winner for that hole. During play a reckoning of the holes is kept by saying that one player or side is so many "holes up" (ahead on the score) or "all square" with so many holes left to play. Accordingly, a player or side can win the match when they are up by one more hole than the number of holes left to play.

The more common method of scoring is stroke play, whereby players simply record the number of strokes taken for each hole and then tabulate the total for the round. The winner is the player having taken the fewest total strokes.

ON THE TEE

● There are two meanings for the word "tee." One is the peg on which the ball is set to elevate it off the ground. The other is the starting place for each hole, properly called the "teeing ground," but almost always simply called the tee. In accordance with the rules, the ball may only be teed on the tee. (It cannot be pegged anywhere except on the teeing ground.)

● On the teeing ground there will be two markers. To start each hole, the ball must be set between the two markers, or no more than two club-lengths behind them.

● If you tee up the ball and it falls off the tee or is accidentally knocked off when you are addressing it, the ball may be replaced without penalty. But if you swing at the ball and miss, a stroke must be counted. (This applies, also, to any other time or place when you swing at the ball and miss.)

● Suppose you swing at the ball and just manage to nick it enough to trickle it off the tee, but it still lies on the teeing ground. Can you set it back up on the tee again? Nope! The next shot must be played from the ground as it lies.

- The player who had the lowest score on the previous hole is said to have the "honor" and shall be the first to hit from the tee. The other players then hit according to their scores, lowest to highest. How is this determined for the first hole of the course? Simply by agreement of the players. And what if two or more players tie for the lowest score on the previous hole? It then reverts back to who had the honor on the hole preceding.

PLAYING THE BALL

- After the ball has been hit from the tee, it must be played as it lies for each shot. Sometimes an exception is made for the so-called "winter rules," which is an allowance for players to improve the lie of their ball when a course is not in top playing condition. Essentially it permits a repositioning of the ball when it lies in a rut, a bare spot, a tire track, or anything else that is not intended to be a natural or designed hazard of the course, or when weather conditions have made the fairways unsatisfactory. This allowance is **not**, however, recognized in the official rules of golf and therefore can be granted **only** by the management of a particular course, who will usually post a sign indicating when such play is allowed.

- The player who is farthest from the hole should always be the next to play.

- Any attempt to strike the ball at any place on the course must be counted as a stroke, even if you completely miss the ball.

- At anyplace other than on the tee, if you accidentally move the ball, even if it's during your address or preliminary waggle, you must count a stroke and play the ball as it lies.

- Suppose your ball lies in the rough. Can you remove any vegetation to get a better path for your swing? You cannot disturb anything that's **growing**. But you can move loose, natural impediments such as tree branches, fallen leaves, loose stones, and the like. But if you move the ball while doing this, there's a two-stroke penalty. (Or a loss of hole in match play.)

- You may also, at any time, move artificial obstructions such as a water hose, refuse container, bench, or anything else that would interfere with your swing. However, if it's an immovable artificial obstruction, such as a drinking fountain, sprinkler head, shelter, etc., the ball may be lifted and dropped within one club-length of the nearest point of relief from the obstruction, but no nearer to the hole, without penalty.

- Whenever a ball may be dropped in accordance with the rules, you must stand erect, face any direction, hold the ball at shoulder height and arm's length, and simply drop it. If it strikes you or your equipment or comes to rest further than two club-lengths from the point of drop, or if it rolls into a hazard or out-of-bounds, the ball must be re-dropped. But you can never drop the ball so it lands closer to the hole than its original lie.

- If a shot of yours finishes on the wrong putting green, the ball must be removed and dropped off the green within one club-length of the nearest point of relief, but not nearer the hole. There's no penalty.

- What if your ball lies on a paved cart path? The cart path is considered to be an immovable obstruction, and therefore the ball may be dropped elsewhere, but no nearer the hole. However, walls, fences, stakes, railings, or anything else that defines out-of-bounds are not immovable obstructions, and no relief is allowed without penalty.

Suppose your ball **does** lie up against a boundary marker, or next to a tree, or some other equally bad spot, what now? You must decide whether you can play it from there, and if so you must play it as it lies. If you decide you cannot play the ball, you may go back to the spot from which you originally hit the ball to play another, and add a one-stroke penalty to your score for the hole. Or, also with a one stroke penalty, you may drop the ball within two club lengths of the point where the ball lay or **any distance** behind that point on a direct line away from the hole.

Anywhere on the course, except in a hazard or on a putting green, if your ball lies in or touches casual water (a temporary accumulation of water not intended to be a hazard of the course), you may remove the ball and drop it within one club-length of the nearest point of relief. This allowance is also granted if the casual water interferes with your stance or swing, or when the ball lies in ground under repair, or in a hole made by a burrowing animal that prefers a golf course for its home. In these cases, there is no penalty for removing the ball and dropping it as the rules allow.

You are the sole judge of whether the ball is playable or not. You may actually declare an unplayable lie at any time on the course (except when the ball is in a water hazard), but if you do so for any reason other than the no-penalty circumstances described above, you must always be willing to accept a one-stroke penalty for lifting the ball and dropping it elsewhere.

There is no penalty (except on the green) if your ball strikes another player's, and you may at any time request another player to mark and move their ball when it obstructs your play.

BALL OUT OF BOUNDS

Out of bounds is that area, usually marked by a fence, stakes, or other obvious boundary, where play is disallowed. Probably the most common, albeit often unwitting, violation of the rules occurs when a ball leaves the course to go out of bounds or into a water hazard. The rules state that you must now play another ball from the spot where you hit the original ball. This is the "stroke-and-distance" penalty, whereby you must charge yourself a penalty stroke for having hit out of bounds, and you also lose the distance the original ball carried. However, most players will walk to the site where their ball actually left the course and play the next ball from there. This is understandable and even tacitly condoned, owing to crowded course conditions and the accent on speedier play. But the subsequent accounting error is unforgivable. Unless you go back to the original spot from where the ball was hit to take the stroke-and-distance penalty, the correct assessment is **two strokes** when you play the next shot from where the ball went out of bounds.

A ball is considered lost if it cannot be found within five minutes after beginning the search for it. In this case the correct accounting is, again, a stroke and-distance penalty. The "acceptable" decision is to play the next ball from an in-bounds position approximating where the lost ball was presumed to be, with a **two-stroke** penalty.

If you discover your "lost" ball after you have put another ball into play, you must continue to play with the second ball, and you must keep the two-stroke penalty (or the stroke-and-distance penalty if that response was employed).

If you hit a shot that you think may have gone out of bounds, to save time you may hit a **provisional ball** from the same spot, provided you do so before going forward to look for the ball, and you inform your opponent of your intentions.

If you have hit a provisional ball and later find that your original ball did not go out of bounds, you must pick up the provisional ball and play the original ball. There is no penalty incurred. If the original ball is indeed out of bounds, you must add a penalty stroke and continue playing with the provisional ball. In this second case you have, by playing the provisional ball, honored the "distance" of the stroke-and-distance penalty.

● BALL IN HAZARD

There are two kinds of hazards: bunkers and any body of water. When the ball is in either one, loose impediments may not be moved, but it is permissible to move artificial objects, such as the rake, that is often found lying in a bunker. Or, if the ball in a bunker is not visible because it's covered by sand, or fallen leaves, etc., you may remove as much of the material as is necessary to see the top of the ball. There is no penalty if you move the ball while doing this, although it must be replaced to its original spot.

When playing from a bunker or water hazard, you may not let your club touch the sand or water before your swing. Penalty for a violation (it's called "grounding" the club) is two strokes or loss of hole in match play.

If you hit a ball into a water hazard, you do **not** need to take a stroke-and-distance penalty as you do when hitting out of bounds. You may instead drop a ball, under penalty of **one** stroke, at any distance behind the hazard, keeping the point where the ball entered the water between you and the hole. If this is impossible to do because the water hazard runs laterally to the hole, you may drop within two club-lengths of the point where the ball entered the water, incurring the one-stroke penalty.

If, in a bunker, your ball lies in casual water or ground under repair, you may lift it without penalty and drop the ball **in the bunker** as near to the original lie as possible, but not nearer the hole. Or you may drop the ball outside the bunker at any distance along a direct line from the hole through the original lie, but not nearer the hole, and for this privilege you must add one stroke to your score.

If you are certain your ball has been lost, in-bounds, in ground under repair, or in casual water, or in a hole made by a burrowing animal, you may drop and play another ball without penalty.

● ON THE PUTTING GREEN

On the green, if your ball is in (or the path of-your putt will take the ball through) casual water or any other unnatural condition of the green, you may lift the ball without penalty and **place** it at the nearest point of relief, but not nearer the hole.

Sand and loose soil are considered loose impediments on the green (along with things such as fallen leaves or branches) and may be removed or brushed aside. If the ball is accidentally moved in doing this, it shall be replaced, without penalty.

There is a two-stroke penalty or loss of hole if you touch the green in your line of putt, except that you may do so to remove loose impediments or repair damage to the green (such as from a ball or spiked shoes), or to set your club in front of the ball as part of your preparatory stance.

⚇ If your putt strikes an unattended flagstick you must take a two-stroke penalty or lose the hole. This is, surprisingly, even true if the flagstick has been removed from the hole and is lying on the ground.

⚇ Is there a penalty for striking the flagstick when you hit your shot from off the green? No, even if the ball is putted from off the green.

⚇ If you hit from off the green and your ball finishes against the flagstick but has not dropped into the hole, it cannot be counted as being in the cup. However, you may move or pull the flagstick out, and if the ball then drops into the hole, it is counted as "holed out."

⚇ If your ball, when played from the green, moves another player's ball, that player must replace it to its original spot, and you incur a two-stroke penalty. In match play, however, there is no penalty for striking another ball, although the struck ball must be replaced.

⚇ On the green, the ball may be lifted and cleaned, without penalty, and replaced at the spot from where it was lifted.

⚇ In match play you may concede your opponent's putt at any time. But in stroke play there is no such thing as a conceded putt (called a "gimme").

⚇ You may not make a putting stroke from a stance astride, or with either foot touching the line of the putt or an extension of that line behind the ball.

⚇ When any part of the ball overhangs the hole, you may, after walking to the hole without delay, wait for ten seconds. If the ball then drops it is considered as "holed out." If not, it is considered to be at rest, and must be struck again to hole out.

Equipment

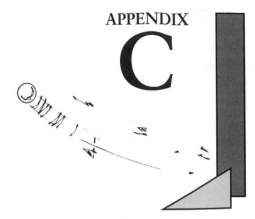

It was once believed unlucky, and unkempt, to play golf in trousers that touched the ground. This led to the long-standing tradition of wearing knickers as common golfing attire, a habit still observed in some areas of Scotland. But the standard apparel for the golfer of today is ordinary slacks and a sporting top. The biggest factor is comfort, and this has evolved into an acceptance on public and almost all private courses of shorts for both women and men, although the "accepted length" is below the fingertips.

Golf is a walking sport, so comfort in footwear is a major consideration. Often, economics is the overruling factor; thus on public courses athletic shoes are common, but the spiked golf shoe is much preferred by experienced players. They provide one with the sure footing of a solid stance, a security especially welcome on full swings and uneven lies.

A specialty item is the golf glove, worn on the left hand; never on both. It melds the hand to the club like instant adhesive, providing against a twisting of the club in the grip from the torque of impact. Why not wear a glove on the right hand? Because that hand gives touch to the swing; direct contact with the club provides a better sense of feel.

THE CLUBS

Sometimes beginning players will purchase, for their first weapons of play, a "starter set" of clubs. This normally includes a one-wood and three-wood, the 3, 5, 7, and 9-irons, and a putter. These clubs will be adequate for most situations on the course, but they limit the development of any player's game. To have complete command over the ball, a full set of clubs will eventually become a necessity.

For tournament play, the rules limit players to a maximum of fourteen clubs. Touring pros sometimes will carry only two woods, nine fairway irons (numbers 1 through 9), a pitching wedge (which has the loft equivalent of a 10-iron), a sand wedge (with a loft even greater than a pitching wedge) and a putter. But the pros hit irons accurately. Amateur players usually hit more reliably when woods are substituted for some of the low irons. Consequently, standard full sets of clubs include a 1, 3, and 5-wood, the numbers 3 through 9-irons, a pitching wedge, and a putter. A 2-wood has become obsolete and a 4-wood uncommon. The 5-wood has replaced the 2-iron in the standard set, and a 7-wood is frequently substituted for a 3- or 4-iron. All this is because the well-engineered woods of today are more manageable in the swing and will provide more accurate results (particularly in higher grass) than the longer, low-numbered irons.

Add a matching sand wedge to your set. It is often considered to be the best stroke-saving club in the bag. It's not only for sand. It can be a perfect club for short approach shots and close-in recoveries from heavy rough or for high lob shots that you want to settle onto the green.

Most sets of irons do not include a sand wedge. Choose one that will match your other irons, or at least avoid those which are heavy or have a bulky flange. They are difficult to control and will feel strangely different in your hands from the rest of your irons. Try to obtain a sand wedge with a rounded leading edge rather than a straight edge. It will slide through the sand instead of digging too deeply, and, when used on a side slope, it will deliver the clubface more squarely into the ball.

Some players even carry a third wedge, with a loft of about sixty degrees (a pitching wedge normally is fifty to fifty-five degrees). This extreme lofted club allows for a full swing on close-in shots, which for many players is easier to execute than a half-swing.

Be sure you have a driver. It's not uncommon to find players with a neurotic fear of the driver, but this is usually because they have not developed enough confidence in its power potential. Typically, the driver is needed on fourteen of the eighteen holes.

Lie of the clubs

One general consideration for all clubs is their lie. That's how the club sits on the ground when you hold it in your normal stance. The blade should sit mostly on the heel, with the toe up about two degrees. This will compensate for the normal twisting of the club during the swing and will actually deliver the clubface into the ball at a proper alignment.

Length

Does it mean that to obtain a correct lie, tall players need longer clubs? Possibly. But it depends, actually, on how far your fingertips are from the ground. Thus, to be properly fitted with clubs of suitable length, make your purchase at a store that specializes in golf equipment. They will custom fit the clubs after seeing not only your normal address posture but also your swing. Generally, better players handle longer clubs more effectively than beginning players.

Grips

Basically, grips are available in leather and rubber composition. Best criterion? How the grip feels in your hands. Another criterion? Cost, because leather grips are considerably more expensive. Besides, there are rubber composition grips available that look and feel remarkably like leather. And they have better gripping ability since they feel "tackier" in your hands; thus they are less likely to twist during the swing. Moreover, leather is less practical in northern climates because in cooler weather the grip can feel too rigid and is especially brutal on off-center hits.

Fit yourself with a grip of proper circumference. Wrap your left hand around the club, three-quarters of an inch from the end of the handle. Your fingertips should gently touch the heel of your hand.

Head

The business end of the club has undergone considerable change in design and construction over the years, particularly the woods. Formerly, the heads of woods were laminated layers of wood (some are still available), but now almost all woods have heads of cast metal. As a result, there is a consistent quality to their manufacture. This also provides the distinct advantages of being less expensive and virtually damage-proof. They are so durable that all they'll ever need, in time, is new grips.

Both woods and irons today offer a larger effective hitting area (called the sweet spot). This is because of perimeter weighting, whereby the clubhead is designed to have a proportionally greater percentage of its weight around the outer edges of the hitting surface, effectively expanding the area where optimal force can be transmitted to the ball. The benefit is that on off-center hits the ball will still acquire good distance with less probability of deviant flight.

Shaft

In the early part of a forceful downswing, the shaft of the club experiences a natural backward bend, then recoils for contact with the ball. The common belief is that a stiff shaft will supply a livelier "snapping" action during this recoil and the ball will thus be given greater distance. It has led to the great majority of players improperly choosing a shaft that is too stiff for their swing. The problem is that a stiff shaft requires a powerful swing to bend it back for an effective recoil, and this generally means being able to produce a clubhead speed of 100 miles per hour or more. Although the shafts today are lighter and the necks smaller to reduce air resistance, the average recreational player seldom generates a clubhead speed exceeding ninety miles per hour. Consequently, a medium-flex shaft is often a more appropriate choice. All this supports, once again, the logic of having a professional analyze your swing before a purchase.

Swing Weight

Basically, the swing weight of a club is the proportion of its head weight to its length. The trend has been toward lighter shafts, with a greater share of the total weight of the club in the head, where it will impart more weight

directly behind the ball at impact. But for some players a head-heavy club could feel like swinging a rock on the end of a string. So the best test is how the club feels in your hands when swung.

The Putter

The lonely putter. It's the only club that never gets used for a full swing, and thus manufacturers seldom try to match it to the rest of the clubs; yet it may be the most important weapon.

There's a dazzling array of choices available. What are some factors to narrow the choice? In general, a heavier putter will help in swinging the clubhead back and through the ball with a slower stroke, which is an advantage if you're having trouble with consistency. And, an offset blade (where the blade is behind the shaft) will help you to keep your hands properly positioned at address. In fact, an offset blade may the most important criterion for beginning players. There's a tendency, in the early stages of acquiring putting skill, to be "wristy" in the stroke; but an offset blade will help to keep the hands ahead of the ball and the clubhead square at impact.

Be sure to select a putter with a proper lie. Never anticipate that you will adapt your putting posture to suit the characteristics of the club. Instead, take enough time to find a putter that is configured for your normal style.

In the final analysis, then, club choices are a matter of personal fit. Suitable clubs depend on how fast you normally swing, how much strength you put into your swing, the arc of your swing, even your stance, and other factors that are best analyzed by a professional. Just as you would seek medical advice from someone trained, go to pro shops or golf specialty stores for advice on club selection. Golf is their only business. They will fit you with clubs that complement your playing characteristics. There are no good clubs or bad clubs, only bad combinations of player and clubs.

▌● THE BALL

And then there is the object of all this attention — a mere 1.62 ounces of a spheroid. It must be manufactured within strict specifications, although there is an allowance for differences in compression. That's a number — 80, 90, or 100 — that indicates how quickly the ball will regain its shape when it's compressed, and thus its liveliness. A 100 compression ball is potentially livelier, and should therefore have greater distance capability. But that's true only if the ball can be compressed upon clubhead impact; otherwise it will not absorb as much kinetic energy and will actually be less responsive. A high-compression ball is, in effect, harder, with more resistance to compression.

Therefore its distance potential is available only to big hitters who can effectively flatten the ball on the clubhead.

The best measure of performance for a ball is, strange as it may seem, how the ball *feels* and *sounds* when you hit it. There is actually not enough difference in the distance potential of high- or low-compression balls to use that as a factor for purchase. Rather, the swing characteristics of your clubs and the quality of force you generate at the moment of impact will determine the distance and accuracy of the resulting shot. So try different compressions, and from different manufacturers. A ball that does not respond well to your own swing will feel like a hunk of lead when you hit it and you'll hear a "thunk" at impact. A ball that is lively off your club will provide you with the feedback of a solid hit and a higher-pitched "thwack" at impact.

A Short History

Somewhere in time, someplace on a bleak Scottish moor, a bored shepherd boy began swatting a whittled ball of boxwood from one rabbit hole to another. Was this the unassuming start of golf?

More glamorous accounts have attempted to trace the game to a pastime called "paganica," which was known to the soldiers of ancient Rome and was carried by them to Britain. But their diversion was obscure and cannot accurately be held as the origin of golf. It has also been suggested that golf originated in France, with a game called "jeu de mail," and this too was transported to Britain. But the French game was more like croquet. In the fifteenth century the Dutch apparently did play a game on frozen canals called "kolf," and it was imported by mercenary soldiers to their homeland of Scotland. But "kolf" was really ice hockey. Besides, the Scots were known to have been playing a golf-like game for decades before the Dutch game arrived. So maybe it really was the shepherd boy who brought his sheep in from their summer pasture and told his friends, "Ye wanna heer oov tha game Ah've invented?"

This much is certain: The Scots were the first to use a variety of clubs to knock a ball over a prescribed course toward a hole in the ground. Iron-faced clubs were in use possibly as early as 1420. It is known that this sporting endeavor became so popular that in 1457 King James ll forbade the playing of the game because it was distracting from the more important matter of archery, which was necessary for defense of the country. But the Scots continued in their pursuit of golf as an alternative to invading England.

The first courses in Scotland were laid out on the dune country by the sea, where the hazards were all natural growths of grass or happenstance scatterings of rocks. The Scots could have been the first to vent their frustration over these hazards by tossing their clubs, for primitive golf clubs have been found on the sea bottom as far as a mile from shore.

Initially, play on the courses-by-the-sea was random, starting at some convenient spot and shooting toward some arbitrary target. Eventually the courses assumed prescribed boundaries, although the number of holes depended on the space available. Legend has it that the standard of eighteen holes for a course was decreed by a golfing authority in Scotland who found that his ever-present flask would be emptied of its golden liquid after eighteen holes of play.

Ultimately golf became so popular in Scotland that it was decided the game needed a basilica in the stature of Notre Dame de Paris or the Great Mosque of Lahore. Thus was established the Royal and Ancient Golf Club of St. Andrews, today an hour's drive northeast of Edinburgh. The course is probably the oldest in the world, having been in continuous play since at least 1754, the date of its earliest records. The sovereignty of St. Andrews is well known. Golfers make a pilgrimage there to step on the immutable turf that is the acknowledged center of the golfing universe.

In America, golf may have been played in the colonies as early as the seventeenth century, but the first specific reference is not found until 1779, as an advertisement for golf balls in a New York newspaper. There are other early newspaper announcements of golfing activities — one in Charleston, South Carolina, in 1795, and another in Savannah, Georgia, in 1796 — but it is believed that these were essentially social clubs rather than active golf clubs.

Other than these brief notices, little is known about golf in the United States until 1884, when a group of West Virginia enthusiasts, most of whom were Scots, formed the Oakhurst Golf Club, generally regarded as the first true golf organization in the country. They built a nine-hole course near White Sulphur Springs, but the game did not gain popularity in the area and the course was soon abandoned.

The first organized golf club to find longevity began in 1888 in Yonkers, New York, and was aptly named the St. Andrews Club. But surprisingly, the first eighteen-hole course did not open until 1893, in Chicago. Thereafter golf grew rapidly. By 1900 there were approximately 400 courses in the United States, and by 1925 there were over 4,500. Most of the first courses were private, but with the Depression there was a general takeover by city and county governments, and consequently public courses became

more common. Thus the game was more available for everyone, and its popularity flourished. Today, there are at least 14,000 (this includes private, public, and par-3) courses. An, there are about fifteen million people who play at least fifteen rounds of golf per year.

The oldest of all golf tournaments, the British Open, was first held in 1860 at Prestwick, Scotland. The first U.S. Open was held at the St. Andrews course in Yonkers in 1894. One year later the first ladies' tournament was inaugurated.

When it became apparent that players could actually make a living playing golf, the Professional Golfers' Association of America (the PGA) was founded in 1916. It was soon followed by the LPGA, the Ladies Professional Golf Association.

Although golf has now penetrated to virtually every corner of the world, it still remains most closely associated with the United States and Britain. This is reflected in the fact that all major tournaments are held in these countries, and together they administer the rules and regulations that govern the play of golf all over the world.

Who are some of the players that have been recognized, over the years, as the greatest ever? Perhaps the question is answered by the original roster of players inducted into the World Golf Hall of Fame. This museum opened in 1954 in Pinehurst, North Carolina. Its first list of golfing greats included only thirteen names: Patty Berg, Walter Hagen, Ben Hogan, Bobby Jones, Byron Nelson, Jack Nicklaus, Francis Ouimet, Arnold Palmer, Gary Player, Gene Sarazen, Sam Snead, Harry Vardon, and "Babe" Zaharias (who has been recognized as the greatest woman athlete of this century).

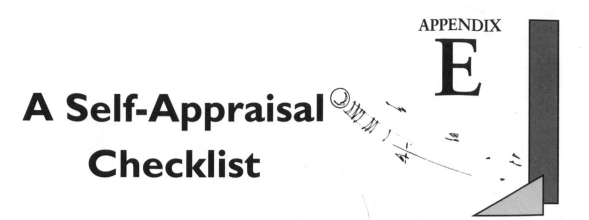

A Self-Appraisal Checklist

What follows here is a series of reminders about the essentials of each aspect of golf. They are cues which may help to set off the right muscle patterns — small packages of information to remind your body of the things it ought to be doing.

Check the appropriate box for each item on the list, or have someone else evaluate your performance. Use the checklist as a reference, noting those parts of your game which appear to need improvement, then orient your practice time around those factors.

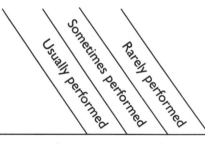

PERFORMANCE CUES

	Usually performed	Sometimes performed	Rarely performed
For every swing:			
1. Position the club across the palm of your left hand, but in the fingers of your right hand.			
2. Stay relaxed, yet alive, limber, and responsive.			
3. Set up so the ball is at the bottom of your swing arc.			
4. Be natural in your stance. Do not exaggerate any aspect of it. Distribute your weight evenly.			
5. Stay in motion before the swing. No static halt to your address routine.			
6. Bring the club into the backswing as a unit, arms and hands together. Make it a one-piece takeaway.			

	Usually performed	Sometimes performed	Rarely performed
7. Start slowly. Gain momentum throughout the swing.			
8. Keep a steady head through the whole swing.			
9. Swing like the club is part of you — a literal extension of your arms.			
10. Keep your arms relatively extended for the whole swing.			
11. Make every stroke fluid, free-flowing, rhythmical.			
12. Keep the club alive — active through contact. Emphasize the follow-through.			
13. Let your swing be dynamic, lively, expressive.			
14. Make the whole motion continuous, with no hesitations.			
15. Enjoy the sensory stimulus of the game itself.			

To hit for power:

1. Get full extension into the windup. Coil into a good shoulder turn.			
2. Take a wide swing arc. Let the left arm be the radius of the arc.			
3. Be loose before the swing. No tension in the arms. No stiffness in your body.			
4. Unweight your front foot as you coil into the backswing.			
5. Transfer the weight forward for the downswing. At contact almost all the weight is on the front foot.			
6. Coil into the backswing with the upper body, but start the uncoil into the downswing with the lower body.			
7. Accelerate the clubhead through contact. Do not be tentative. Explode into the ball.			
8. Imagine you are carrying the ball forward on your clubhead as you contact it.			

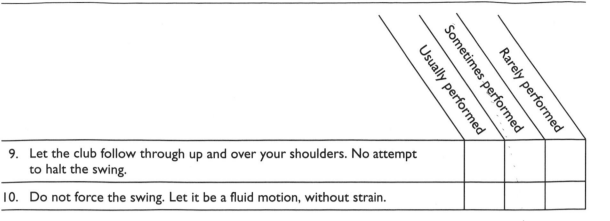

	Usually performed	Sometimes performed	Rarely performed
9. Let the club follow through up and over your shoulders. No attempt to halt the swing.			
10. Do not force the swing. Let it be a fluid motion, without strain.			

When chipping the ball:

1. Make sure you have selected the right club for the situation.			
2. Set up close to the ball. Open the stance and the clubface.			
3. Choke down on the club, and set hands ahead of clubhead.			
4. Select an aim point, on the green if practical, and focus on that point.			
5. Program the distance of the shot by the length of your backswing.			
6. Make the swing an arm motion, with minimal body rotation.			
7. Keep the wrists steady for the swing.			
8. Stay unhurried, but fluid and rhythmical.			
9. Sweep club over top of grass. Hit through the ball, not under it.			
10. Take a positive strike at the ball. No tentativeness.			

When pitching the ball:

1. Use trees, flagstick, etc., to aid in judging the needed distance.			
2. Find and appropriate landing point for the ball.			
3. Rehearse the swing before the final setup.			
4. Adjust the setup according to the distance needed (open stance and forward hands for closer shots).			
5. Keep the club in acceleration through impact.			
6. Use more body rotation and weight shift for longer shots.			

	Usually performed	Sometimes performed	Rarely performed
7. Take a smooth swing, with a follow-through that is not consciously halted.			
8. When pitching the ball high, use active wrists.			
9. For a pitch and run, have hands well forward and keep wrists steady through impact.			
10. Always account for both flight and expected roll of the ball in selecting the aim point.			

On the putting green:

1. Read the green as you approach it, noting the overall lay of the surface.			
2. Have a consistent pre-shot routine of judging the line of the putt, rehearsing the swing, and final setup.			
3. Keep palms aligned parallel with the putter blade.			
4. Have a solid, balanced base for the setup.			
5. Make the swing an arm-dominated pendular motion.			
6. Keep a quiet head and steady body for the whole stroke.			
7. Keep a consistent bend in the left elbow through contact.			
8. Take a deliberate backswing, but without hesitancy.			
9. Guide the club with the left hand; push it forward with the right.			
10. Swing with the same pace and rhythm for all putts; vary the distance by the length of the backswing.			

From the sand:

1. Open both club and stance, at equal angles.			

	Usually performed	Sometimes performed	Rarely performed
2. Pick spot in sand. Focus intently on that spot. Bring club into the spot. Do not hit ball directly.			
3. Hit firmly. Bring club convincingly through the sand.			
4. Do not attempt to scoop the ball or chop the club into the sand.			
5. Finish the swing with a high follow-through.			

Other trouble spots:

	Usually performed	Sometimes performed	Rarely performed
1. From the rough, use more of an upright swing, and more wrists.			
2. To stay low under branches, lay hands well forward; keep wrists firm, and hit punch shot.			
3. To go over trees, release wrists fully as you come into the ball.			
4. On uphill or downhill lie, align weight with hill. Stay steady for the swing. Bring club path parallel with the slope.			
5. When ball is below feet, stand close to ball, with extra bend in knees and waist.			
6. When ball is above feet, set weight on toes, stand tall.			

As strategy for the course:

	Usually performed	Sometimes performed	Rarely performed
1. Never rush the opening drive.			
2. Keep the ball in play, always allowing for a margin of error.			
3. Take the safest route to the green.			
4. Target the ball to hit away from potential trouble areas.			
5. Plan ahead. Consider not only the immediate shot, but also what the result will be for the next shot.			

	Usually performed	Sometimes performed	Rarely performed
6. Always focus on a specific target. Don't be overconscious of lurking trouble. Attend only to the point of aim.			
7. Always use enough club to reach your objective.			
8. Play only the shots you are capable of making. Stay within your ability.			
9. Use your natural flight character by allowing for it instead of fighting against it.			
10. Always consider the percentage of potential success in planning the shot.			

As states of mind:

	Usually performed	Sometimes performed	Rarely performed
1. Self-talk optimism into your mind. Believe in your own ability.			
2. Maintain a state of calm, even after having hit a poor shot.			
3. Focus on each shot. Forget the previous shot. Play each ball as if it were the only one you will hit that day.			
4. Believe that every ball will go where you want it to.			
5. Visualize the flight of the ball before you take your swing.			
6. Use visualization often, not only before every shot, but also as mental rehearsal during quiet, non-playing times.			
7. Always hit for a positive target instead of cautiously trying to steer the ball away from trouble.			
8. Keep an upbeat attitude, and competitive spirit, for the entire round.			
9. Compete against the course, not against an opponent.			
10. Find enjoyment in the very act of playing.			

Index

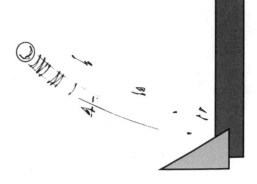